Abdominal/GI Emergencies

Editors

SARA MANNING
NICOLE McCOIN

EMERGENCY MEDICINE CLINICS OF NORTH AMERICA

www.emed.theclinics.com

Consulting Editor
AMAL MATTU

November 2021 • Volume 39 • Number 4

ELSEVIER

1600 John F. Kennedy Boulevard • Suite 1800 • Philadelphia, Pennsylvania, 19103-2899

http://www.theclinics.com

EMERGENCY MEDICINE CLINICS OF NORTH AMERICA Volume 39, Number 4
November 2021 ISSN 0733-8627, ISBN-13: 978-0-323-83590-9

Editor: Joanna Collett
Developmental Editor: Axell Ivan Jade Purificacion

Emergency Medicine Clinics of North America (ISSN 0733-8627) is published quarterly by Elsevier Inc., 360 Park Avenue South, New York, NY, 10010-1710. Months of issue are February, May, August, and November. Business and Editorial Offices: 1600 John F. Kennedy Boulevard, Suite 1800, Philadelphia, PA 19103-2899. Customer Service Office: 6277 Sea Harbor Drive, Orlando, FL 32887-4800. Periodicals postage paid at New York, NY, and additional mailing offices. Subscription prices are $100.00 per year (US students), $359.00 per year (US individuals), $926.00 per year (US institutions), $220.00 per year (international students), $462.00 per year (international individuals), $986.00 per year (international institutions), $100.00 per year (Canadian students), $423.00 per year (Canadian individuals), and $986.00 per year (Canadian institutions). International air speed delivery is included in all *Clinics'* subscription prices. All prices are subject to change without notice. **POSTMASTER:** Send address changes to *Emergency Medicine Clinics of North America*, Elsevier Periodicals Customer Service, 11830 Westline Industrial Drive, St. Louis, MO 63146. Customer Service (orders, claims, online, change of address): Elsevier Periodicals **Customer Service, 11830 Westline Industrial Drive, St. Louis, MO 63146. Tel: 1-800-654-2452 (U.S. and Canada); 314-453-7041 (outside U.S. and Canada). Fax: 314-453-5170. E-mail: journalscustomerservice-usa@elsevier.com (for print support); journalsonlinesupport-usa@elsevier.com (for online support).**

Reprints. For copies of 100 or more of articles in this publication, please contact the Commercial Reprints Department, Elsevier Inc., 360 Park Avenue South, New York, NY 10010-1710. Tel.: 212-633-3874; Fax: 212-633-3820; E-mail: reprints@elsevier.com.

Emergency Medicine Clinics of North America is covered in *MEDLINE/PubMed (Index Medicus), Current Contents/Clinical Medicine, EMBASE/Excerpta Medica, BIOSIS, SciSearch, CINAHL, ISI/BIOMED,* and *Research Alert.*

Contributors

CONSULTING EDITOR

AMAL MATTU, MD, FAAEM, FACEP
Professor and Vice Chair of Academic Affairs, Department of Emergency Medicine, University of Maryland School of Medicine, Baltimore, Maryland

EDITORS

SARA MANNING, MD
Assistant Professor, Department of Emergency Medicine, Indiana University School of Medicine, Indianapolis, Indiana

NICOLE McCOIN, MD
Chair of Emergency Medicine, Ochsner Medical Center, New Orleans, Louisiana

AUTHORS

DANIEL S. BRENNER, MD, PhD
Assistant Professor, Department of Emergency Medicine, Indiana University School of Medicine, Indianapolis, Indiana

ALEXIS L. CATES, DO
Attending Physician, Division of Medical Toxicology, Department of Emergency Medicine, Einstein Healthcare Network, Philadelphia, Pennsylvania

KRISTI COLBENSON, MD
Assistant Professor, Emergency Medicine and Sports Medicine, Mayo Clinic, Rochester, Minnesota

KEVIN M. CULLISON, MD
Clinical Assistant Professor, Ronald O. Perelman Department of Emergency Medicine, NYU Grossman School of Medicine, New York, New York

LIZA DILEO THOMAS, MD, CPXP, FAAEM, FACEP
Assistant Clinical Professor, Department of Emergency Medicine, Ochsner Medical Center, New Orleans, Louisiana

SAHAR MORKOS EL HAYEK, MD
Instructor of Emergency Medicine, Washington University in St. Louis, St Louis, Missouri

BRENNA FARMER, MD, MBA, MS
Vice Chair, Quality and Patient Safety, Associate Professor of Clinical Emergency Medicine, Department of Emergency Medicine, Weill Cornell Medicine, Site Director, NewYork-Presbyterian/Lower Manhattan Hospital Emergency Department, New York, New York

TIFFANY C. FONG, MD
Assistant Professor, Department of Emergency Medicine, Johns Hopkins School of Medicine, Baltimore, Maryland

NATHAN FRANCK, MD
Clinical Instructor, Ronald O. Perelman Department of Emergency Medicine, NYU Grossman School of Medicine, New York, New York

MAGLIN HALSEY-NICHOLS, MD
Associate Program Director, The University of North Carolina at Chapel Hill, Chapel Hill, North Carolina

MEGAN C. HENN, MD, FACEP
Assistant Professor, Department of Emergency Medicine, Emory University, Atlanta, Georgia

ELIZABETH LEENELLETT, MD
Department of Emergency Medicine, University of Cincinnati, Cincinnati, Ohio

ZACHARY BERT LEWIS, MD
Assistant Professor of Emergency Medicine, University of Arkansas for Medical Sciences, Little Rock, Arkansas

SARA MANNING, MD
Assistant Professor, Department of Emergency Medicine, Indiana University School of Medicine, Indianapolis, Indiana

NICOLE McCOIN, MD
Chair of Emergency Medicine, Ochsner Medical Center, New Orleans, Louisiana

NEERAJA MURALI, DO, MPH
Assistant Professor, Department of Emergency Medicine, University of Maryland School of Medicine, Baltimore, Maryland

SREEJA NATESAN, MD
Division of Emergency Medicine, Duke University Hospital, Durham, North Carolina

BRIAN K. PARKER, MD
Department of Emergency Medicine, Assistant Clinical Professor, UT Health San Antonio, San Antonio, Texas

ADAM RIEVES, MD, MS
Department of Emergency Medicine, Washington University in St. Louis, St Louis, Missouri

DAVID C. SNOW, MD, MSc
Assistant Professor of Emergency Medicine, Loyola University Medical Center, Maywood, Illinois

JOSEPH WESLEY WATKINS IV, MD
Assistant Professor of Emergency Medicine, University of Arkansas for Medical Sciences, Little Rock, Arkansas

ELIZABETH BARRALL WERLEY, MD
Assistant Professor, Department of Emergency Medicine, Penn State Health Milton S. Hershey Medical Center, Hershey, Pennsylvania

CARMEN WOLFE, MD
Assistant Professor, Department of Emergency Medicine, Vanderbilt University Medical Center, Nashville, Tennessee

Contents

The physical examination of the patient is the cornerstone of the practice of medicine, and the skills to complete a thorough abdominal examination are critical in the care of patients. When performed correctly, the abdominal examination can be revealing when it comes to the overall health of the patient as well as acute pathology. The examination of the abdomen has the potential to minimize further testing or radiation and serves as a key diagnostic tool. In this article, we will discuss each portion of the abdominal examination in detail as well as pathologic findings, abdomen-specific signs, special patient populations, and clinical pearls.

Abdominal pain is the most common chief complaint in the Emergency Department. Abdominal pain is caused by a variety of gastrointestinal and nongastrointestinal disorders. Some frequently missed conditions include biliary pathology, appendicitis, diverticulitis, and urogenital pathology. The Emergency Medicine clinician must consider all aspects of the patient's presentation including history, physical examination, laboratory testing, and imaging. If no diagnosis is identified, close reassessment of pain, vital signs, and physical examination are necessary to ensure safe discharge. Strict verbal and written return precautions should be provided to the patient.

Although abdominal pain is a common chief complaint in the emergency department, only 1 in 6 patients with abdominal pain are diagnosed with a gastrointestinal (GI) emergency. These patients often undergo extensive testing as well as hospitalizations to rule out an acute GI emergency and there is evidence that not all patients benefit from such management. Several clinical decision rules (CDRs) have been developed for the diagnosis and management of patients with suspected acute appendicitis and upper GI bleeding to identify those patients who may safely forgo further testing or hospital admission. Further validation studies demonstrating the superiority of these CDRs over contemporary practice are needed.

> Abdominal pain is one of the most common presenting complaints to the emergency department (ED). More often than not, some degree of laboratory testing is used to narrow the differential diagnosis based on the patient's history and examination. Ordering practices are often guided by evidence, habit, consulting services, and institutional/regional culture. This review highlights relevant laboratory studies that may be ordered in the ED, as well as commentary on indications and diagnostic value of these tests.

> Abdominal pain represents 5% to 7% of all emergency department presentations. Many patients require imaging for diagnosis, and choosing the appropriate imaging modality is a crucial decision point. Modern medicine offers a fantastic array of options including abdominal radiograph, computed tomography, MRI, and ultrasonography, but the plethora of alternatives can be paralyzing. This article introduces the commonly available modalities, discusses the advantages and disadvantages, and presents current recommendations for commonly diagnosed conditions.

> Abdominal vascular emergencies are an uncommon entity in emergency medicine, but when they present, they are often catastrophic. These time-sensitive and life-threatening diagnoses are often hidden in nonspecific complaints such as nausea, vomiting, or flank pain, so the emergency physician must remain diligent and consider these in the differential diagnoses. The following is an overview of the more common of these abdominal vascular emergencies, in the hope that they help the Emergency Physician avoid the misdiagnosis and subsequent vascular catastrophe that would follow.

> Postprocedural complications encompass a wide array of conditions that vary in acuity, symptoms, index procedure, and treatment. Continued advancements in diagnostic and therapeutic procedures have led to a significant shift of procedures to the ambulatory setting. This trend is of particular interest to the emergency physician, as patients who develop complications often present to an emergency department for evaluation and treatment. Here the authors examine a high-yield collection of procedures, both ambulatory and inpatient, notable for their frequent utilization

and unique complication profiles including common laparoscopic surgical procedures, bariatric surgery, endoscopic procedures, interventional radiology procedures, and hernia repairs with implantable mesh.

Abdominal pain is a common complaint in the emergency department, comprising 8.8% of all visits. Despite advances in medicine and imaging, 20% to 30% of patients still leave the department without a definitive diagnosis, whichhis can be both distressing for patients and unsatisfying for providers. Diagnoses of exclusion can be perilous, and their application should be carefully considered in order to not overlook more emergent complaints. However, a working knowledge of diagnoses of exclusion can guide therapeutics and specialty referrals that can ultimately provide answers and relief to a patient population often at odds with available information and expectations.

EMERGENCY MEDICINE CLINICS OF NORTH AMERICA

SERIES OF RELATED INTEREST

Gastroenterology Clinics
https://www.gastro.theclinics.com/
Critical Care Clinics
https://www.criticalcare.theclinics.com/

THE CLINICS ARE NOW AVAILABLE ONLINE!
Access your subscription at:
www.theclinics.com

EMERGENCY MEDICINE
CLINICS OF NORTH AMERICA

Foreword

Abdominal and Gastrointestinal Emergencies

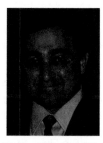

Amal Mattu, MD, FAAEM, FACEP
Consulting Editor

Many clinicians refer to the brain as the "black box" of the human body because brain and other neurologic disorders tend to be difficult to diagnose. However, I would argue that, with due diligence, neurologic disorders can and almost always *should* be diagnosed because they follow simple rules and anatomic pathways. I would instead suggest removing that "black box" label from the brain and affixing it prominently to a patient's *abdomen*.

In my opinion, there is no region of the body that is more perplexing than the abdomen, and no organ system that is more puzzling than the gastrointestinal (GI) system. Abdominal and GI disorders can produce pain in remote areas, such as the chest, back, or pelvis; even when abdominal pain is present, it may occur in atypical locations. Further confounding our efforts at proper diagnosis is the fact that classic abdominal/GI complaints, such as vomiting and diarrhea, often occur in the setting of neurologic, cardiac, urologic, infectious, metabolic, and other disorders. Vital signs and most laboratory studies are neither sensitive nor specific, and the exam itself can be misleading. It is no surprise, therefore, that intra-abdominal disorders account for a significant number of misdiagnoses and malpractice cases in emergency medicine. This relatively high risk of misdiagnosis is present despite the availability of advanced imaging, such as ultrasound and computed tomography. I've always believed that a "master clinician" is one who has mastered the abdomen!

Fortunately, for those of us that still see a black box when we look at the abdomen, Guest Editors Drs Nicole McCoin and Sara Manning have assembled an outstanding group of authors to shed some light on abdominal and GI pathology. This issue of *Emergency Medicine Clinics of North America* begins with an outstanding article focused on "Perfecting the Gastrointestinal Physical Examination" that should be considered mandatory reading for all acute care clinicians. Next is an article that addresses the chief complaint of abdominal pain with a focus on misdiagnoses.

Emerg Med Clin N Am 39 (2021) xiii–xiv
https://doi.org/10.1016/j.emc.2021.08.006
0733-8627/21/© 2021 Published by Elsevier Inc.

emed.theclinics.com

Subsequent articles then take us through the workup, including decision rules, laboratory testing, and imaging. Special scenarios and populations are addressed, including postprocedural GI emergencies, traumatic issues, immunocompromised patients, and those who chronically abuse drugs. Two final articles address abdominal pain mimics and diagnoses of exclusion.

This issue of *Emergency Medicine Clinics of North America* is an outstanding addition to the continuing medical education of acute care providers at every level. I particularly appreciate that the editors and authors did not simply focus on a basic core curriculum by addressing each individual organ, but instead addressed higher-level topics and the needs of experienced clinicians. Kudos and thanks to the contributors for providing a text that is sure to make that abdominal black box brighter and more opaque for us all!

Amal Mattu, MD, FAAEM, FACEP
Department of Emergency Medicine
University of Maryland School of Medicine
110 South Paca Street
6th Floor, Suite 200
Baltimore, MD 21201, USA

E-mail address:
amattu@som.umaryland.edu

Preface

Gastrointestinal Emergencies

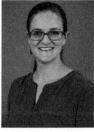 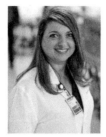

Sara Manning, MD   Nicole McCoin, MD
Editors

Numerous studies have quantified our observed reality on a shift in the emergency department: abdominal pain, nausea, vomiting, diarrhea, and constipation are common, and, at times, the definitive cause of these signs and symptoms is challenging to diagnose. The breadth of conditions that present with abdominal complaints varies widely from the benign to acutely life-threatening; from the clearly gastrointestinal in origin to manifestations of extraintestinal pathologic conditions; from chronic and lingering to rapidly progressive. As such, the emergency medicine clinician's approach to patients with these complaints must be thorough, nuanced, and multimodal.

In this issue of *Emergency Medicine Clinics of North America*, the articles unfold in the same fashion as the emergency medicine clinician's typical approach to the patient with abdominal complaints. The articles start with a focus on the abdominal exam and subsequently transition to sections that follow the thought process of the clinician as the exam concludes and orders are placed. These articles focus on the creation of the differential diagnosis, such as "no-miss" abdominal pain diagnoses, as well as clinical decision rules to guide management. The articles that follow elaborate on laboratory and imaging diagnostics commonly ordered in the workup of abdominal complaints. We then explore specific patient populations and presentations that pose unique diagnostic or treatment dilemmas, including abdominal vascular emergencies, postprocedural abdominal emergencies, occult abdominal trauma, the immunocompromised patient, the patient with chronic drug use, and those patients with conditions of extraintestinal origin who present with abdominal pain. Finally, we wrap up with a discussion of the approach to patients with diagnoses of exclusion.

We commend the authors of this issue of *Emergency Medicine Clinics of North America* on their diligent efforts. Their hard work has resulted in a collection of interesting and thorough reviews that reflect the state-of-the-art in medical management of patients with gastrointestinal emergencies. It is our intent to enrich clinicians with all levels of experience in a variety of practice settings with tools that aid them in the

Emerg Med Clin N Am 39 (2021) xv–xvi
https://doi.org/10.1016/j.emc.2021.08.003
0733-8627/21/© 2021 Published by Elsevier Inc.

workup of abdominal complaints from the beginning to the end of the patient encounter. We hope the content presented here provides a robust understanding of this exceedingly common presenting complaint and allows for efficient, safe, cost-effective care.

Sara Manning, MD
Department of Emergency Medicine
Indiana University School of Medicine
720 Eskenazi Avenue, FOB 3rd Floor
Indianapolis, IN 46202, USA

Nicole McCoin, MD
Ochsner Medical Center
1514 Jefferson Highway
New Orleans, LA 70121, USA

E-mail addresses:
Smanning4@iuhp.org (S. Manning)
Nicole.mccoin@ochsner.org (N. McCoin)

Perfecting the Gastrointestinal Physical Exam

Findings and Their Utility and Examination Pearls

Liza DiLeo Thomas, MD, CPXP, FAAEM, FACEP[a,*],
Megan C. Henn, MD, FACEP[b]

KEYWORDS

- Physical examination • Abdominal • Emergency • Peritoneal signs • Rebound
- Analgesia

KEY POINTS

- The abdominal examination is an essential part of the physical examination of the emergency medicine patient.
- The basic abdominal physical examination can be broken down into different components: inspection/exposure, percussion, auscultation, and palpation.
- Knowing how to perform an excellent abdominal examination can help narrow your differential diagnosis and serve to minimize further testing in the emergency department.
- Sensitivity and specificity for clinical signs varies; a working knowledge of their limitations is necessary to use these signs in daily practice.
- Special populations including children, the elderly, pregnant, and unstable patients pose diagnostic challenges making the abdominal examination more difficult but still useful.

INTRODUCTION TO THE ABDOMINAL EXAMINATION

A complete examination of the abdomen is typically composed of several elements — inspection, percussion, auscultation, and palpation of the abdomen, as well as examination of the head, neck, mouth, and rectum, when indicated. Patient positioning and comfort are critical in achieving a reliable examination.[1] The examination of the abdomen should also include an overall evaluation of the patient. While elderly

[a] Department of Emergency Medicine, Ochsner Medical Center, 1514 Jefferson Highway, New Orleans, LA 70121, USA; [b] Department of Emergency Medicine, Emory University, 531 Asbury Circle, Annex Building, Suite N340, Atlanta, GA 30322, USA
* Corresponding author.
E-mail address: liza.dileothomas@ochsner.org
Twitter: @lzzza3 (L.D.T.); @megan_henn (M.C.H.)

Emerg Med Clin N Am 39 (2021) 689–702
https://doi.org/10.1016/j.emc.2021.07.004
0733-8627/21/© 2021 Elsevier Inc. All rights reserved.

patients can appear well even with life-threatening pathology, an ill-appearing patient with abdominal pain should be urgently evaluated as there are many concerning potential etiologies of their pain.[2] While this part of the examination is only one piece of a thorough history and physical examination, it can reveal much about the patient's general health as well as the acute complaint.

ELEMENTS OF THE ABDOMINAL EXAMINATION
Inspection/Exposure

Before examining a patient, the examiner should obtain consent. After thoroughly washing hands, the examiner should explain to the patient the reason for the examination and the steps that will be involved. Inspection of the abdomen is the beginning of a thorough abdominal examination and should not be omitted as it can reveal a great deal about the patient. The abdomen should be fully exposed from the chest wall to the pubic symphysis, and the patient positioned in a comfortable, supine position allowing for abdominal muscle relaxation,[1] ideally with the knees and head supported.[3] The patient's hands should be at the side or folded across the chest. The visual examination of the shape, skin, color, and movement of the abdomen begins the search for pathology.[3]

The examiner should inspect the skin for color, rash, wounds, scars, and medical equipment, customarily observed from the patient's right side or from the foot of the bed.[3,4] Skin inspection can reveal a great deal about the patient's general health as well as findings that may indicate abdominal pathology. For example, surgical scars or more recent healing incisions, a vesicular rash consistent with zoster, striae indicating possible Cushing's syndrome,[1] bluish discoloration at the umbilicus (Cullen's sign) or the flanks (Grey Turner's sign),[1] dilated abdominal wall veins (**Fig. 1**), or an ostomy or stoma may be present.

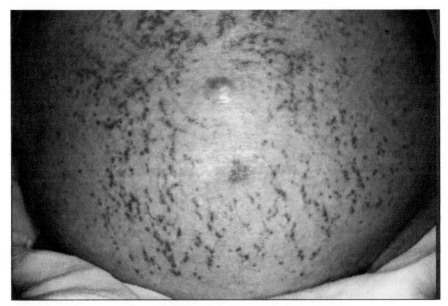

Fig. 1. Stigmata of liver disease. Dilated abdominal wall veins associated with cirrhosis and portal hypertension. (Jackson JM, Callen JP, Greer KE. Dermatological Signs of Systemic Disease. 2017. Page 255-261.)

The examiner should observe the contour and shape of the abdomen. The presence of ascites, a gravid uterus, enlarged abdominal girth, or distention may be appreciated. Visible masses that could indicate hernias (**Fig. 2**), tumors, lymphadenopathy, or infection should also be denoted. Asking the patient to contract the abdominal muscles may provide additional visual clues as muscle tension will make a mass within the abdominal wall more apparent while relaxation of the abdominal wall will make a mass within the abdominal cavity more prominent.[1]

Movement observed in the abdominal wall can include the use of accessory muscles for increased work of breathing, pulsatile masses in the case of an abdominal aortic aneurysm (AAA), or peristalsis indicating a possible bowel obstruction.

Auscultation

The abdominal examination continues with auscultation of bowel sounds. Classic medical textbooks suggest that this portion of the examination usually precedes percussion and palpation because of the possibility of disturbing the bowel sounds during those portions of the examination. However, a randomized controlled trial by Calis and colleagues[5] found that the order of the examination did not change the frequency of bowel sounds. Bowel sounds can be heard best with the use of the stethoscope diaphragm, usually in one location such as the right lower quadrant, as bowel sounds are transmitted throughout the abdomen.[6] The examiner may occasionally hear borborygmi, what we typically describe as the "stomach growling," which corresponds with loud, prolonged sounds of hyperperistalsis.[6] A normal frequency of bowel sounds is every 5 to 10 seconds,[1] and an increase or decrease in frequency of bowel sounds can indicate pathology of the bowels. Bowel sounds may be increased in diarrheal illnesses or early intestinal obstruction. They may be decreased and eventually absent in processes such as ileus and peritonitis.[6] High-pitched tinkling sounds may indicate intestinal obstruction because those sounds may correspond with air under tension in a dilated bowel.[6] However, auscultation of bowel sounds is not altogether reliable and is time-intensive[2] as the examiner must listen for a full 3 minutes to establish that bowel sounds are truly absent.[3] Also, diminished or absent bowel sounds may not be present in intestinal obstruction and is an unreliable indicator of a perforated viscus or other surgical abdomen.[7]

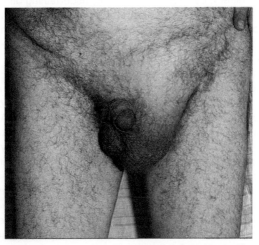

Fig. 2. Inguinal hernia. Left indirect inguinal hernia. (Merritt R, Clyne B. Ferri's Clinical Advisor 2021. Page 799.)

In addition to bowel sounds, the examiner may hear vascular bruits of the renal, iliac, or femoral arteries.[1] If these bruits are heard only in systole, this may be normal and may not indicate occlusive disease. However, if there are both systolic and diastolic components to the bruits, this suggests turbulent blood flow, and therefore, partial arterial occlusion is likely present.[6]

Percussion

Percussion of the abdomen can be used to determine the nature of an abdominal mass and help maximize knowledge of intra-abdominal pathology. In order to appropriately perform percussion, the examiner should place the second or middle finger of the nondominant hand firmly on the area to be percussed and hyperextend it.[6,8] Contacting the area with other parts of the hand, other than this finger, will dampen the vibrations and affect the sound. Then, using the second or middle finger on the dominant hand, tap against the middle finger of the resting hand until a sound is heard. The wrist should be moved in a quick striking movement as though it is bouncing off of the other hand,[6] similar to a piano hammer.[8] The strike should occur just below the nail and with the tip of the finger of the nondominant hand. Tympanitic resonance or tympany is obtained over a hollow body and is usually higher in pitch.[8] Tympany indicates that a mass is gas filled while dullness implies a mass is solid or fluid filled. During abdominal percussion, if tympany is heard over the umbilicus and there is dullness at the flanks, free fluid in the abdomen may be suspected. While the patient lies supine, fluid gravitates to the flanks; therefore, there will be dullness when percussing the flanks and resonance when percussing the epigastric and umbilical regions.[8] The examiner can then check for shifting dullness by having the patient lie on one side, waiting 10 seconds or more, and then percussing from the uppermost flank toward the umbilicus. A change from tympany to dullness indicates that gas has moved to the top and fluid has shifted down to gravity.[4] Without testing for shifting dullness, merely percussing for fluid at the flanks does not conclusively indicate that there is free fluid in the abdomen.[8] Percussion can also be used to determine spleen size and liver size while listening for dullness change to tympany as the examiner's fingers transition from solid organs to gas-filled bowel.

As with each part of the abdominal examination, there are limitations to the value of percussion. The examiner may have more difficulty ascertaining difference in sound in patients with an elevated body mass index or those who have edema to the abdominal wall.[8] Also, in critically ill patients or those in severe pain, the examiner may need to defer this part of the examination.

Palpation

Palpation of the abdomen with the intent to identify and localize pain is one of the most useful elements of the abdominal examination. Palpation of the abdomen should be completed with the patient supine and as comfortable as possible. As mentioned previously, the head and knees should be supported to allow the abdominal wall muscles to relax. The examiner should palpate the abdomen twice — initially superficially, followed by deep palpation to examine each quadrant of the abdomen (**Fig. 3**).

To begin this portion of the examination, the examiner should describe this portion of the examination and its purpose to the patient. To perform the examination, typically the examiner stands to the right side of the patient.[4] The examiner's hands are ideally warm and fingernails are short. If necessary, the examiner may make contact with the patient through the gown if the examiner's hands are cold.[6] The patient can indicate the area of most intense pain and, if there is a focal area, that area should be palpated last, after palpating the rest of the abdomen.[8] Palpation should be performed by

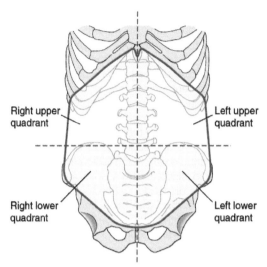

Fig. 3. Quadrants of the abdomen. (*From* Joanna Kotcher Fullerb. Surgical Technology – Principles and Practice, 8th edition. Chapter 22 – General Surgery, Fig. 22.2 (caption: *The quadrants of the abdomen*).)

keeping the fingers together and flat against the abdominal surface while the hand and forearm are on the same plane as the supine patient and gliding the hand across the abdomen smoothly while gently dipping into all quadrants. While moving across the abdomen, the examiner should monitor the patient's facial expressions while both palpating and lifting the hand off the skin just slightly.[6] This superficial palpation will reassure and relax the patient while allowing for discovery of areas of tenderness and irregularities that can be further explored on deep palpation.

One objective of palpating the abdomen is to localize and quantify tenderness. Describing the pain in reference to its location, depth, and severity can reveal much about the patient's intra-abdominal pathology. The patient may avoid pain by contracting the abdominal wall musculature. This contraction is referred to as guarding. Guarding can be voluntary, where the abdominal wall muscle is contracted to avoid palpation of the intra-abdominal contents,[3] or involuntary. Involuntary guarding is a spasm of the abdominal wall that is not controlled by the patient and often indicates peritoneal inflammation. Raising the knees and head as well as relaxing the patient can often decrease voluntary guarding.[3] As previously mentioned, the patient's arms should be at the side or crossed over the chest. The arms should not be rested above the head, as this will stretch and tighten the abdominal wall.[6] Relaxation techniques, such as asking the patient to take a few deep breaths with the jaw dropped open[6] or by attempting to distract the patient with conversation, may help the examiner determine whether the guarding is voluntary or involuntary.

Deep palpation will follow superficial palpation and is necessary to assess the presence of abdominal masses and to further assess the location, character, and quality of the pain. Palpation should again be performed with the palmar surfaces of the fingers throughout all four quadrants. Once masses are identified, their location should be noted, as well as their size, shape, consistency, tenderness, pulsations, and mobility.[6] In patients with muscular resistance, obesity, or abdominal wall edema, deep palpation is better accomplished using two hands. Usually, the dominant hand is placed on top of the nondominant hand, with the upper hand placing pressure and the lower hand focusing on palpation.

While superficial palpation already identified the concerning areas of tenderness, with deep palpation, the examiner may be able to further localize the tenderness and determine if there is peritoneal irritation. The patient may have indicated that coughing or simply moving on the bed worsens the abdominal pain. If not, the examiner can ask the patient to cough, and if the cough produces pain in a specific location, this is likely an area of localized peritoneal irritation.[6] The examiner can also now check for rebound tenderness. Rebound tenderness can be described as worsening pain on release of deep palpation. It results from movement of the inflamed peritoneum. It is performed by pressing the fingers into the region of concern slowly and firmly to depress the peritoneum for 15 to 30 seconds and then release the fingers quickly from the skin.[9] The examiner should watch and listen closely for signs from the patient that this maneuver has elicited discomfort.[6] A positive finding of rebound is established if the patient experiences discomfort when the fingers were released. The patient should indicate where the pain was most intense during the examination. If tenderness was felt in a location other than where the examiner was palpating, that area may be the source of peritoneal irritation.[6]

Patients with diffuse peritonitis, which may occur in perforated viscus cases such as a perforated ulcer, perforated appendicitis, perforated diverticulitis, or even in patients with acute pancreatitis, will sometimes be described as having a "boardlike" or rigid abdomen.[3] This is due to involuntary guarding that is present in these cases. Otherwise, the location of tenderness can usually help narrow the differential. In terms of gastrointestinal sources, right upper quadrant tenderness frequently indicates biliary disease, ulcer disease, hepatitis, or pancreatitis. Epigastric tenderness may indicate pancreatitis or peptic ulcer disease. Right lower quadrant tenderness may be due to acute appendicitis, perforated carcinoma, or cecal diverticulitis. Left lower quadrant tenderness is usually secondary to sigmoid diverticulitis.

Palpation of the abdomen will also allow the examiner to determine other abnormalities such as crepitus of the abdominal wall, which indicates air in the subcutaneous tissue.[4] Crepitus in the abdominal wall is introduced either by trauma or by infection from gas-producing bacteria.[3]

Digital Rectal Examination

While classically the digital rectal examination (DRE) was considered to be a critical portion of the abdominal examination, the utility of the DRE is limited. DRE can be a useful screening tool in the setting of anorectal, urologic, or gynecologic pathology but does not provide diagnostic guidance in most intra-abdominal pathologies. Specifically, the use of DRE to determine the need for surgical intervention in the setting of possible acute appendicitis has not proven to be accurate and may lead to inappropriate surgical management.[10]

However, classic teaching is that the abdominal examination ends with the DRE. If the examiner determines that a DRE is indicated, the procedure will need to be thoroughly explained to the patient, and consent should be obtained. With an appropriate chaperone, but still maintaining the patient's privacy, a lubricated, gloved finger should be placed against the patient's rectal sphincter muscle to relax it, then slowly moved into the rectum while palpating for any masses or foreign bodies.[4] While prostatitis typically presents with urinary symptoms, it can be a cause of lower abdominal and, in particular, suprapubic pain.[11] The examiner should palpate the prostate for tenderness or bogginess, which can indicate prostatitis.[4] A rigorous digital prostate examination should be avoided in these patients as it can lead to systemic bacteremia.[11] After the finger is removed, the glove should be visually inspected for blood or melena.[4]

Genitourinary Examination

The utility of the pelvic examination in the evaluation of abdominal pain has been debated as studies cite few cases where the management plan changes based on the examination, and the examination itself can be unreliable.[12,13] Often difficult to complete in the emergency department because of space and privacy restraints and found to be a poor test with low sensitivity,[12] the pelvic examination has more recently been discussed as an unnecessary part of the examination of a patient with abdominal pain. However, although the pelvic examination can be an invasive examination for your patient, there may be findings that can significantly impact the patient's management plan. One study examined the utility of pelvic examinations with the goal to look for adnexal tenderness, cervical motion tenderness, uterine tenderness, uterine bleeding, discharge, and abnormalities of the cervical os and found that 6% (12/183 patients) had findings that were unexpected and changed the clinical plan.[13] These aforementioned findings can suggest diagnoses associated with significant morbidity and mortality including ovarian pathology, pelvic inflammatory disease, uterine masses, cervicitis, and malignancies.

Testicular examinations, searching to evaluate specifically for an abnormal testicular lie, high riding testicle, or absence of the cremasteric reflex, should be included in your examination of the male patient with abdominal pain to rapidly evaluate for testicular torsion.[14] Skin changes on the ipsilateral scrotum may be present including induration, erythema, and warmth as an indicator of prolonged inflammation.[15] An abnormal examination is only reported in 50% of patients with testicular torsion,[14] but if torsion is suspected, surgical intervention should not be delayed for further imaging diagnostics.[15] If the diagnosis is unclear based on history and examination, then scrotal ultrasound with Doppler should follow immediately.[15]

SIGNS AND TESTS

Table 1 shows the most common physical examination maneuvers as well as their respective sensitivities and specificities.

Other tests, while commonly performed, have less robust data regarding their sensitivity and specificity in the evaluation of a patient with abdominal pain. These are listed in the following paragraphs.

Caput Medusa

In hepatic cirrhosis, inspection of the abdominal wall can reveal caput medusa, the descriptive term given to distended veins flowing away from the umbilicus.[4]

Carnett's Sign

Anterior cutaneous nerve entrapment is a case where abdominal pain can fool the examiner into thinking there may be a deeper, visceral cause of the pain. Carnett's sign is used to differentiate between an intra-abdominal cause of pain versus abdominal wall pain. If this sign is present, straight leg raise or another maneuver that tenses the abdominal wall musculature will worsen the patient's abdominal pain, or palpation of the area during this maneuver worsens it. This indicates that the pain is localized to the abdominal wall.[18]

Closed Eyes Sign

Patients with an organic disease causing abdominal pain usually leave their eyes open while the examiner performs an abdominal examination, while those patients with nonspecific abdominal pain will close their eyes.[19]

Table 1
Abdominal signs on physical examination[16,17]

Sign	Disease Process	Description	Sensitivity	Specificity
Rovsing	Acute appendicitis	Pressing the hand deeply in the left lower quadrant results in pain at McBurney's point.	19%–75%	58%–93%
McBurney	Acute appendicitis	When applying pressure at McBurney's point (1.5–2 inches from the anterior superior iliac spine on an imaginary line drawn to the umbilicus) with one finger, pain is elicited.	83%	45%
Psoas	Acute appendicitis	The examiner asks the patient to lie on the opposite side (left) and extend the leg on the affected side (right). Extension of this leg will cause pain. The examiner may also place pressure against the patient's knee while they attempt to raise it. Alternatively, the patient may also hold the hip in flexion to relieve pain. These maneuvers stretch the psoas muscle which is painful in an inflamed appendix but also can be painful in the setting of a psoas abscess, urologic, or paraspinal condition.	13%–42%	79%–97%
Obturator	Acute appendicitis	The examiner stands on the right of the patient and slightly flexes the right thigh, to relax the psoas muscle. Then the limb is internally rotated at the hip. Test is positive if the patient complains of hypogastric pain with this movement.	8%	94%
Murphy	Acute cholecystitis	The patient is unable to take a full inspiration while the examiner is palpating deeply underneath the costal margin in the right upper quadrant.	48%–97%	48%–96%

Cullen's Sign

Cullen's sign is periumbilical ecchymosis. This indicates intra-abdominal or retroperitoneal hemorrhage.[4]

Grey Turner's Sign

In hemorrhagic pancreatitis, patients can develop ecchymosis of the flanks and groin known as Grey Turner's sign.[4]

SPECIAL CONSIDERATIONS
The Unstable Patient

The obtunded, intubated, or otherwise critically ill patient is often unable to provide a thorough history. Unfortunately, the physical examination also lacks reliability in this clinical scenario, introducing the risk of diagnostic errors.[20] The most common infectious etiology in critically ill patients is intra-abdominal pathology, but the physical examination only aids in the diagnosis 42% to 69% of the time in the setting of intra-abdominal abscess.[20] While adjunct testing becomes critical to accurately diagnose possible intra-abdominal sources of the illness, many of these patients are not stable enough to undergo testing or imaging. Aggressive resuscitation is often needed, and the early administration of broad-spectrum antibiotics should be emphasized. While diagnostic imaging, most commonly computerized tomography, plays an important role in the evaluation of the critically ill patient, the physical examination directs the plan of care in choosing the correct imaging modality and location.[20]

Pediatric Population

The pediatric population poses several diagnostic challenges because of the limited history based on the verbal development of the child, caregiver involvement, as well as the wide spectrum of pediatric-specific gastrointestinal diseases. Especially in the preverbal or young child, the caregivers may be the best source of historical information. The age of the child often determines the utility of the history in addressing the pediatric patient with abdominal pain. With a limited history, the examination becomes all the more critical in the evaluation of younger patients. The positioning of the child and introduction of the examiner in a nonthreatening way is the first step in eliciting reliable results from the examination.[9] In talking with the patient first, allowing the child to remain in the caregiver's lap, and starting with painless components of the examination, the examiner will develop trust of the child and elicit a more reliable examination.[9] Distraction techniques of talking, using the stethoscope for palpation, or examining the abdomen during sleep can all be useful tools in examining the abdomen of an anxious pediatric patient.[9] In addition to the aforementioned examination method of detecting rebound tenderness to indicate peritoneal inflammation, other maneuvers in children may be helpful. Asking the patient to jump up and down, bumping the bed, or tapping the feet may elicit discomfort in the abdomen consistent with peritoneal pain, similar to rebound tenderness.[9]

Elderly Population

As our society ages, so does the emergency department patient population. Geriatric patients frequently require special attention as they are prone to worse outcomes, higher rates of hospital admission and surgical intervention, and longer emergency department (ED) and hospital stays than our younger patients.[21] Elderly patients are more likely to present with diffuse and nonspecific pain and have a more subtle presentation, and therefore, they will require a more time- and resource-intensive evaluation.[22] There are several reasons why geriatric patients are unique. Physiologic changes occur to almost every organ system as the patient ages, and this can affect not just the patient's presentation but also the response to interventions.[22] Typical findings of rebound and guarding may be absent because of atrophy of abdominal wall musculature.[21] Changes in the peripheral nervous system may change the perception of pain and may lead to a more subtle presentation and even a delay of the patient's presentation to the ED. This patient population is more likely to be on medications that may interfere with or blunt the physical examination, such as steroids, beta-blockers, nonsteroidal anti-inflammatories, or opioids.[21,22] In patients older than 80 years, mortality more than doubles if the diagnosis is missed[21]; therefore, the examiner must remain cognizant of the limitations of the geriatric patient's physical examination and maintain a high index of suspicion of significant intraabdominal pathology.

Pregnant Population

This special patient population has a wide variety of anatomic and physiologic changes that occur during pregnancy and vary by gestational age, and determining the cause of acute abdominal pain in these patients can be difficult. After 12 weeks of gestation, the uterus becomes an abdominal organ and can begin to compress the abdominal viscera.[23] The abdominal wall also becomes more lax which can delay findings of peritoneal signs.[23]

The most common reason for nonobstetric surgical intervention in pregnant patients is appendicitis, which affects 1 in 1500 pregnancies. Traditional teaching is that the appendix rises in the peritoneal cavity as the uterus enlarges, beginning around 12 weeks, reaching the iliac crest around 24 weeks. However, more recently, this has been challenged.[23] A high clinical suspicion is necessary when evaluating these patients because morbidity is high. An unruptured appendix has a fetal mortality rate of 3% to 5%, while a ruptured appendix has a fetal mortality rate of 20% to 25% and 4% maternal mortality.[23] These mortality rates are significant when compared to the overall mortality rate of appendicitis, which is 0.27% to 0.29% for unperforated and 1.18% for perforated.[24,25] Not only are peritoneal signs delayed in pregnant patients but the location and character of their tenderness also differ from those of the nonpregnant patient. Biliary disease is another cause of abdominal pain in pregnant patients as it is thought that the increase in sex steroids during pregnancy causes delayed gallbladder emptying. However, acute cholecystitis is not more common during pregnancy. Physical examination findings of acute cholecystitis are similar to those in the nonpregnant patient with right upper quadrant tenderness and possibly a positive Murphy's sign.[23]

Although the abdominal examination is a critical portion of the physical examination and reveals a great deal of pathology in the patient, there are limitations that may make the abdominal examination less reliable. Pregnancy can obscure landmarks, especially in later gestational ages. In addition to the anatomic changes in pregnancy, the decreased tone in abdominal wall muscles can decrease the ability to detect rebound tenderness. This change can also be seen in elderly patients. In addition, obesity, abdominal ascites, psychiatric disease, and intoxication can decrease the reliability of the abdominal examination. Other chronic disease processes including diabetes and chemotherapy or steroid-induced immunosuppression can alter the examination findings.

OTHER/ADJUNCTS TO THE ABDOMINAL EXAMINATION

A complete evaluation of the patient should take place in addition to the abdominal examination described previously. These adjuncts to the abdominal examination

Table 2
Adjuncts to abdominal examination[4]

Location	Finding	Possible Disease Process
Arms/hands		
Limbs	Asterixis/tremor	End-stage liver disease/alcohol withdrawal
Arms	Track marks (scarring over veins)	Possible intravenous drug use (past or present)
Limbs	Dialysis fistula/graft	End-stage renal disease
Hands/feet	Pallor	Anemia
Face/neck		
Eyes	Scleral icterus	End-stage liver disease
	Pallor of conjunctiva	Anemia
	Kayser-Fleischer ring (due to excess deposition of copper)	Wilson's disease
	Xanthelasma (periorbital lipid deposits)	Chronic cholestasis
Mouth/oral cavity	Oral ulcers	Crohn's disease, celiac disease
	Angular cheilitis	Iron deficiency
	Red, beefy, smooth tongue	Vitamin B-12, folate deficiency
	Fruity odor to breath	Diabetic ketoacidosis
Neck	Virchow's node (supraclavicular lymph node)	Gastric or breast cancer

can complete the clinical picture and give indicators to the pathology affecting the patient. In **Table 2**, we describe specifics in the remainder of the examination and how it may correlate with abdominal pathology.

CLINICAL CONTROVERSIES AND MYTHS
Is it possible to detect an abdominal aortic aneurysm (AAA) on physical examination? Is it safe?

AAAs are often asymptomatic and contribute to a significant number of potentially preventable deaths in the United States yearly. Once ruptured, the AAA has a mortality rate of almost 50%.[26] One cost-effective way to detect an AAA is by abdominal palpation[27] (**Fig. 4**). The palpation of an AAA to measure the width can be a highly sensitive way to evaluate for an AAA large enough to indicate the need for surgical intervention with a sensitivity of 72% of AAA measured at 4 cm or larger.[27] However, body habitus can decrease that sensitivity (91% vs 53% sensitivity with abdominal girth >100 cm).[26,27] This physical examination finding of a widened abdominal aorta should be followed by ultrasound to confirm the suspicions found during examination.[27] Although some may worry that it is possible to precipitate a rupture by palpating the aortic pulsation, this has never been reported. Therefore, palpation of the aneurysmal aorta appears to be safe.[28]

Will Giving Pain Medications Mask Important Findings?

Although some may be hesitant to treat patients with pain medication lest it masks signs of a surgical abdomen. Specifically, classic teaching warns us that if patients are given pain medication, consultants, namely surgeons and radiologists, may not appreciate the same examination that the emergency medicine physician has

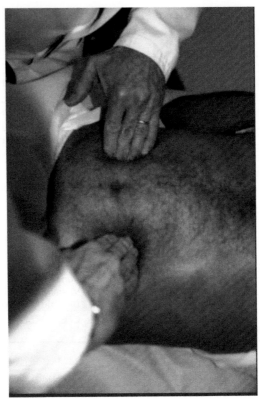

Fig. 4. Inguinal hernia. Estimating an aortic aneurysm diameter as the distance between the closest fingers. (Beckman JA, Creager MA. Vascular Medicine: A Companion to Braunwald's Heart Disease. 2020. Page 474-482.)

obtained. Studies have indicated that this is not the case. Emergency medicine and surgical studies alike have demonstrated that the administration of analgesics does not impair the diagnostic accuracy of examination findings.[29,30] In particular, the sonographic Murphy's sign is not hindered by administration of opioid analgesia.[31]

SUMMARY

Despite the increased use of adjunct imaging, the physical examination remains an informative and necessary part of patient care that gathers information critical to medical decision-making. Here, we have summarized the various components of the abdominal examination including inspection and exposure, percussion, auscultation, and palpation. When carried out correctly, the abdominal examination is a key diagnostic tool and a window into the overall health and acute pathology of the patient.

CLINICS CARE POINTS

- The positioning of the patient is the key to a thorough and accurate examination. The examiner must take the time to explain the examination and place the patient in a comfortable position for a reliable and informative examination.

- A complete abdominal examination includes inspection, percussion, auscultation, palpation, as well as examination of the oral cavity, genitalia, and anus when appropriate.
- Adjuncts to your abdominal examination can provide evidence of intra-abdominal pathologies including examination of the arms, hands, face, neck, and skin.
- There are several signs that can be pathognomonic when examining the patient and that can immediately inform next steps in management.
- Special populations including patients who are pregnant, critically ill, or at the extremes of age may harbor significant intra-abdominal pathologies despite an unremarkable examination.

DISCLOSURE

The authors have nothing to disclose.

REFERENCES

1. Bilal M, Voin V, Topale N, et al. The clinical anatomy of the physical examination of the abdomen: a comprehensive review. Clin Anat 2017;30:352–6.
2. Macaluso C, McNamara R. Evaluation and management of acute abdominal pain in the emergency department. Int J Gen Med 2012;5:789–97.
3. Ferguson CM. Inspection, auscultation, palpation, and percussion of the abdomen. In: Walker HK, Hall WD, Hurst JW, editors. Clinical methods: the history, physical, and laboratory examinations. 3rd edition. Boston: Butterworths; 1990. Chapter 93.
4. Mealie CA, Ali R, Manthey DE. Abdominal exam. In: StatPearls. Treasure Island (FL): StatPearls Publishing; 2020. Available at: https://www.ncbi.nlm.nih.gov/books/NBK459220/.
5. Çalış AS, Kaya E, Mehmetaj L, et al. Abdominal palpation and percussion maneuvers do not affect bowel sounds. Turk J Surg 2019;35(4):309–13.
6. Bates B. A guide to physical examination and history taking. 5th edition. Pennsylvania: J.B. Lippincott Company; 1991. p. 244–6, 339-368.
7. Staniland JR, Ditchburn J, De Dombal FT. Clinical presentation of acute abdomen: study of 600 patients. Br Med J 1972;3(5823):393–8.
8. Cabot R. Physical diagnosis. 11th edition. Baltimore: William Wood & Company; 1935. p. 160–78.
9. Bundy DG, Byerley JS, Liles EA, et al. Does this child have appendicitis? JAMA 2007;298(4):438–51.
10. Sedlack M, et al. Is there still a role for suspected appendicitis in adults? AJEM 2008;26:359–77.
11. Touma NJ, Nickel JC. Prostatitis and chronic pelvic pain syndrome in men. Med Clin North Am 2011;95:75–86.
12. Close RJ, Sachs CJ, Dyne PL. Reliability of bimanual pelvic examinations performed in emergency departments. West J Med 2001;175(4):240–5.
13. Brown J, Fleming R, Aristzabel J, et al. Does pelvic exam in the emergency department add useful information? West J Emerg Med 2011;12(2):208–12.
14. Schmitz D, Safranek S. Clinical inquiries. How useful is a physical exam in diagnosing testicular torsion? J Fam Pract 2009;58(8):433–4.
15. Sharp VJ, Kieran K, Arlen AM. Testicular torsion: diagnosis, evaluation, and management. Am Fam Physician 2013;88(12):835–40.

16. Rastogi V, Singh D, Tekiner H, et al. Abdominal physical signs and medical eponyms: physical examination of palpation part 1, 1876-1907. Clin Med Res 2018;16(3–4):83–91.
17. Rastogi V, Singh D, Tekiner H, et al. Abdominal physical signs and medical eponyms: movements and compression. Clin Med Res 2018;16(3–4):76–82.
18. Hidalgo DF, Phemister J, Ordoñez AC, et al. Carnett's sign: an easy tool that saves unnecessary expenses in the evaluation of chronic abdominal pain. Am J Gastroenterol 2017;112:S760–1.
19. Gray DW, Dixon JM, Collin J. The closed eyes sign: an aid to diagnosing non-specific abdominal pain. Br Med J 1988;297:837.
20. Crandall M, West MA. Evaluation of the abdomen in the critically ill patient: opening the black box. Curr Opin Crit Care 2006;12:333–9.
21. Leuthauser A, McVane B. Abdominal pain in the geriatric patient. Emerg Med Clin North Am 2016;34(2):363–75.
22. Sanson TG, O'Keefe KP. Evaluation of abdominal pain in the elderly. Emerg Med Clin North Am 1996;14(3):615–27.
23. Kilpatrick CC, Monga M. Approach to the acute abdomen in pregnancy. Ob Gyn Clin North Am 2007;34(3):389–402.
24. Peltokallio P, Tykkä H. Evolution of the age distribution and mortality of acute appendicitis. Arch Surg 1981;116(2):153–6. https://doi.org/10.1001/archsurg.1981.01380140015003.
25. Lulchev D. Smŭrtnostta pri ostŭr apenditsit–analiz na desetgodishen period [Mortality in acute appendicitis–an analysis of a ten-year period]. Khirurgiia (Sofiia) 1996;49(6):11–6.
26. Karkos CD, Mukhopadhyay U, Papakostas I, et al. Abdominal aortic aneurysm: the role of clinical examination and opportunistic detection. Eur J Vasc Endovascular Surg 2000;19(3):299–303.
27. Fink HA, Lederle FA, Roth CS, et al. The accuracy of physical examination to detect abdominal aortic aneurysm. Arch Intern Med 2000;160(6):833–6.
28. Lederle FA, Simel DL. The rational clinical examination. Does this patient have abdominal aortic aneurysm? JAMA 1999;281(1):77–82.
29. Gallagher EJ, Esses D, Lee C, et al. Randomized clinical trial of morphine in acute abdominal pain. Ann Emerg Med 2006;48(2):150–60.
30. Gavriilidis P, de'Angelis N, Tobias A. To use or not to use opioid analgesia for acute abdominal pain before definitive surgical diagnosis? a systematic review and network meta-analysis. J Clin Med Res 2019;11(2):121–6.
31. Nelson BP, Senecal EL, Hong C, et al. Opioid analgesia and assessment of the sonographic Murphy sign. J Emerg Med 2005;28(4):409–13.

Abdominal Pain in the Emergency Department
Missed Diagnoses

Maglin Halsey-Nichols, MD[a],*, Nicole McCoin, MD[b]

KEYWORDS

- Abdominal pain • Return visits • Missed appendicitis • Missed cholecystitis
- Missed diagnosis • Emergency department discharge instructions

KEY POINTS

- Abdominal pain is the most common chief complaint and frequent reason for return visits in the Emergency Department.
- Common missed diagnoses in patients presenting with abdominal pain include gastrointestinal as well as nongastrointestinal disorders.
- The Emergency Medicine clinician should consider the full clinical presentation, including history, physical examination, laboratory and imaging studies, as well as response to rendered treatment, to appropriately formulate and narrow the differential diagnosis for the patient with abdominal pain.
- Thorough reassessments, clear follow-up plan, and return precautions are imperative for safe discharge.

INTRODUCTION

Abdominal pain is the most common presenting chief complaint in the Emergency Department (ED).[1,2] The anatomic complexity of the abdomen as well as the frequently overlapping symptom profiles of many conditions creates risk for misdiagnosis. In addition, available resources in the ED, including laboratory and imaging studies, cannot always identify a specific underlying diagnosis. Owing to the multitude of potential diagnoses and limits of ED testing, it is not surprising that this symptom is a major source of return visits and medicolegal cases for both academic and community hospitals.[3–7]

Disclosure: The authors have nothing to disclose.
[a] University of North Carolina at Chapel Hill, Houpt Building (Physician Office Building) Suite 1116, 170 Manning Drive- CB-7594, Chapel Hill, NC 27599-7594, USA; [b] Department of Emergency Medicine, Ochsner Medical Center, 1514 Jefferson Highway, New Orleans, LA 70121, USA
* Corresponding author.
E-mail address: maglin_halsey@med.unc.edu

Emerg Med Clin N Am 39 (2021) 703–717
https://doi.org/10.1016/j.emc.2021.07.005
0733-8627/21/© 2021 Elsevier Inc. All rights reserved.

FACTORS ASSOCIATED WITH MISSED DIAGNOSES
Most Commonly Missed Diagnoses

As evidence of the limitations of ED resources to adequately diagnose etiologies of abdominal pain, some of the most common diagnoses provided at discharge are re-statements of the patient's presenting complaint or attempts at a catch-all diagnosis[1,4,8,9]:

- Abdominal pain/nonspecific abdominal pain
- Nausea and vomiting
- Gastroenteritis
- Other gastrointestinal disorders.

Knowing that abdominal pain is a frequent cause of return visits to the ED, these initial diagnoses are likely being given to patients who have underlying pathology for which treatment may be indicated.

Frequently missed diagnoses and reasons for return visits include both surgical and medical diagnoses. The most frequently noted diagnoses are appendicitis and biliary pathology.[3,4,8]

Other frequently missed diagnoses and causes for return visits include:

- Diverticulitis[3]
- Small bowel obstruction[3]
- Urinary tract infections (UTIs) or urinary retention[3,8,9]
- Ectopic pregnancy[3]
- Cancer[3]
- Other extra-abdominal (especially pulmonary and urogenital) pathologies.[9]

Patient Factors

Although specific patient characteristics do not guarantee the presence or diagnosis of certain conditions, factors exist that may help the EM clinician identify higher-risk populations. Several studies have identified similar factors associated with return visits to the ED for abdominal pain in general[4,6]:

- Older age
- Male
- African American ethnicity
- Medicare/Medicaid insurance.

Additional groups associated with missed diagnosis are patients who have fewer prior ED visits and patients with no history of substance abuse.[3] Other historical features associated with missed diagnoses include right upper quadrant pain, nausea and vomiting, and known comorbidities.[8]

Provider Factors

The clinician has the responsibility of collecting an accurate history and examination, choosing appropriate testing, interpreting the data, pursuing additional workup as indicated, determining treatment, and instructing the patient in appropriate follow-up and return precautions. Herein lies multiple instances where missed diagnoses can occur. One study found that the most common errors involved history-taking, ordering of diagnostic tests, and inappropriate or absent follow-up of test results.[3]

Over half of ED patients with abdominal pain undergo diagnostic testing including serum studies, urine studies, and imaging.[1] The clinician must use a combination of knowledge of the utility of the test and clinical gestalt to determine how and to what degree that test aids in decision making regarding the diagnosis and further workup. For example, a white blood cell count (WBC) is frequently obtained in the workup of abdominal pain. An elevated WBC demonstrates poor specificity; however, in some studies, its presence is associated with missed diagnosis.[6,8] More than any diagnostic study, computed tomography (CT) is the test associated with identifying specific diagnoses in patients presenting with abdominal pain. Early CT imaging improves diagnostic accuracy and may decrease return ED visits.[6,10,11] Still one study noted that 10% of patients initially evaluated in the ED for abdominal pain with a CT subsequently underwent repeat CT imaging within 1 month with 30% showing a new or worsening process.[12] CT imaging still misses diagnoses and has associated cost, radiation exposure, and potential for increased ED length of stay.

COMMON MISSES: GASTROINTESTINAL

There are many abdominal pain diagnoses stemming from disorders of the gastrointestinal system that can present atypically and, if missed, can be associated with significant complications. Diverticulitis, bowel obstruction, bowel perforation, and hernia are a few important examples. As noted earlier, appendicitis and biliary disease are the most commonly missed abdominal pain diagnoses.

Appendicitis

The lifetime risk of appendicitis is between 7% and 9%.[13] Although the classic presentation of findings such as anorexia, low-grade fevers, abdominal pain migrating to the right lower quadrant, and elevated inflammatory markers is often seen, establishing the diagnosis can be quite challenging. In fact, clinical signs or positive laboratory indicators may be absent in up to 55% of cases.[13] It is difficult to establish the proportion of missed diagnoses of appendicitis, but it has been reported, based on insurance claims data, that up to 6% of cases are missed in the initial ED visit.[10] Missed or delayed diagnosis can give rise to significant complications including abscess formation, perforation, and sepsis. Appendicitis is of particular interest to the emergency physician as it is a common, potentially challenging and high-risk diagnosis that is frequently associated with litigation against ED physicians, with claims paid to patients in up to a third of cases.[14]

Regarding the history and physical, the diagnosis of appendicitis is more likely to be missed in women, patients with comorbid conditions, and patients presenting with complaints of constipation.[10] The sensitivity of fever in the diagnosis of appendicitis is approximately 70%, with specificity of 65%. In a meta-analysis of 570 patients with suspected appendicitis, history of fever only yielded a likelihood ratio of 1.64. The diagnostic significance of fever did increase on serial examination.[14] Although lack of tenderness in the right lower quadrant and absence of rigidity or guarding make appendicitis less likely, there were also no findings on clinical examination that can effectively rule out appendicitis.[15]

The WBC is not a specific marker as it is commonly elevated in patients with other inflammatory conditions that may be on the differential for abdominal pain. A WBC limit of greater than 10 to 12,000 cells/mm^3 had a sensitivity of 65% to 85% and a specificity of 32% to 82% in the diagnosis of appendicitis.[14] A 2003 meta-analysis of 3382 patients from 14 studies showed a sensitivity and specificity of a WBC greater than 10,000 cells/mm^3 of 83% and 67%, respectively, with a positive and negative likelihood ratio of 2.52 and 0.26, respectively. The WBC alone only alters the probability of diagnosis of appendicitis to a modest degree and should not be used in isolation to rule in or rule out the diagnosis.[14]

C-reactive protein (CRP) levels show an increase between 8 and 12 hours after the onset of appendicitis with a peak between 24 and 48 hours, which is later than that of the WBC.[14]

A CRP cut-off of greater than 10 mg/L yielded a range of sensitivity between 65% and 85% and a specificity between 59% and 73%. Although the CRP is a strong predictor for appendiceal perforation, it has limited use in the diagnosis of appendicitis, particularly early appendicitis.[14]

The utility of a polymorphonuclear leukocyte (PMN) count (normal adult range 1.8–7.7 $\times$ 10^9 cells/L) in the diagnosis of appendicitis has also been studied. In fact, a 2003 meta-analysis showed that a PMN count greater than 11 $\times$ 10^9 cells/L had a greater likelihood ratio than any other laboratory marker studied in the workup of appendicitis. However, for the likelihood ratio to reach a clinically significant level, the PMN count had to be quite elevated to greater than 13 $\times$ 10^9 cells/L.[14]

There has been much discussion about the utility of combining findings from the history and physical and/or laboratory markers to aid in diagnostic decision making. Sengupta and colleagues calculated a sensitivity of 100%, a specificity of 50%, and an NPV of 100% when either the CRP was $\leq$10 mg/L or WBC was $\leq$11 $\times$ 10^3 cells/mm3.[15] However, Vaughn-Shaw and colleagues[16] replicated this study and found a sensitivity of 92% to 94% and a specificity of 60% to 64%. The Modified Alvarado Scoring System, and, more recently, other tools such as the Appendicitis Inflammatory Response Score and RIPASA Score were created as risk stratification tools for appendicitis that combine elements of the history and physical with laboratory results.[14,17]

CT with intravenous contrast is the gold standard imaging study for appendicitis in adults. In a 2011 study of 2781 patients, CT had a sensitivity of 98.5% and a specificity of 98%. A 2011 meta-analysis of 28 studies comprising 9330 patients found that the negative appendectomy rate was 8.7% when using CT compared to 16.7% when using clinical evaluation alone.[14] A paucity of intraabdominal fat is the most common reason for a false-negative CT study.[18]

Ultrasound and MRI are discussed as alternatives to CT, particularly when the clinician wishes to avoid the use of ionizing radiation in the diagnostic workup. An ultrasound study in the workup of acute appendicitis carries a sensitivity of 83.7% and a specificity of 95.9%.[14] MRI is most commonly discussed in pregnant patients, and, in that population, carries a 91.8% sensitivity and 97.9% specificity for the diagnosis of acute appendicitis.[19]

Cholecystitis

Like appendicitis, cholecystitis carries the combination of frequent occurrence and considerable risk to the patient if missed. Acute cholecystitis typically presents with fever, right upper quadrant pain, and leukocytosis. Female patients and those who are obese are at greater risk. However, once again, atypical presentations are common.

Patients with acute cholecystitis may lack fever. In fact, Gruber and colleagues[20] found 71% of patients with nongangrenous acute cholecystitis and 59% of patients with gangrenous acute cholecystitis were afebrile. Murphy's sign is commonly discussed as a useful physical examination finding in the workup of potential cholecystitis. However, it demonstrates a wide range of sensitivity between 58% and 97%.[21] Furthermore, in the elderly, the sensitivity is even lower. Thus, a negative Murphy's sign alone is not useful in ruling out cholecystitis.[22]

Similarly, WBC is also a poor predictor of acute cholecystitis. Gruber and colleagues demonstrated that 32% of patients with nongangrenous acute cholecystitis and 27%

of patients with gangrenous acute cholecystitis had a normal WBC. Both CRP and the neutrophil-to-lymphocyte ratio have demonstrated improved discriminative power as compared to the WBC.[23,24] Liver function tests may be normal in patients with acute cholecystitis. Padda and colleagues[25] found that only approximately 30% of patients with acute cholecystitis had abnormal alkaline phosphatase and/or bilirubin levels and only approximately 50% had a transaminitis.

The Tokyo Criteria combine clinical, laboratory, and radiographic findings to diagnose and grade cholecystitis. The diagnostic criteria state that either Murphy's sign and/or right upper quadrant mass, pain, or tenderness must be present. In addition, at least one of the systemic signs of fever, elevated CRP, or elevated WBC must be present. Subsequently, imaging findings can confirm the diagnosis. Grades of severity are defined in these criteria based on various examinations and laboratory findings. The criteria were retrospectively reviewed in 445 patients, and increasing grades of severity were linked to increased morbidity.[26]

Classic teaching prescribes the use of ultrasound in the workup of acute cholecystitis. Although the diagnostic yield of ultrasound varies in different studies, it is recommended as the imaging method of choice for this diagnosis as it is not invasive, relatively easy to use, cost-effective, and widely available.[27] CT can be considered in cases in which the differential is broad and the EM clinician is seeking an imaging study that may aid in excluding other nonbiliary diagnoses as well. Interestingly, CT showed an acute nongallbladder abnormality missed during a previous ultrasound in 32% of cases.[28] There are other studies that suggest that cholecystoscintigraphy (HIDA) is a more sensitive test than ultrasound for acute cholecystitis and thus should be potentially considered in the workup of acute cholecystitis in some cases in which there is persistent clinical suspicion after ultrasound.[29]

Summary

A combination of data sources must be used to rule out the diagnoses of appendicitis and cholecystitis. No one laboratory value, physical finding, or imaging study should be used in isolation to exclude the diagnosis. The same applies to other gastrointestinal diagnoses as well. Maintain a low threshold to monitor the patient for some time with serial examinations or involve other health care providers (eg, a surgeon) if the diagnosis remains in question (**Box 1**).

COMMON MISSES: NONGASTROINTESTINAL
Genitourinary

Ovarian and testicular torsion
The most common presenting complaint in patients with ovarian torsion is abdominal pain, which is typically one-sided, most often on the right, and can be intermittent or constant.[30–32] Common associated symptoms include nausea and vomiting.[31,32] This

---

Box 1
Pearls in the evaluation of a patient for a gastrointestinal source of abdominal pain

- Use a combination of data to rule out a gastrointestinal source. An isolated historical point, examination finding, or laboratory value is not sufficient to exclude a diagnosis.

- Maintain a low threshold to involve other health care providers (eg, a surgeon) if the diagnosis in question is one in which delay or lack of diagnosis could be of detriment to the patient and there is still diagnostic uncertainty despite laboratory and radiographic workup.

clinical presentation is similar to other emergent diagnoses, particularly appendicitis. Although patients with ovarian torsion tend to exhibit unilateral abdominal tenderness to palpation, this is not universal.[30] One study in pediatric patients found that anorexia and guarding on abdominal examination were less suggestive of ovarian torsion and more concerning for appendicitis.[31] A palpable adnexal mass is an infrequent but concerning finding for torsion.[31] Laboratory studies usually do not aid in diagnosis, but when comparing to pediatric patients with appendicitis, patients with torsion may have lower WBCs and CRP.[30,31] Ultrasound is by far the most sensitive (79%) imaging study, but a normal ultrasound does not exclude ovarian torsion.[32]

Testicular torsion classically presents with testicular pain, tenderness, and scrotal swelling, but there is a subset of patients who may present with abdominal pain, with one study finding about 22% of pediatric patients with testicular torsion presenting in this manner.[33] Concerningly, clinicians did not consistently perform genitourinary examinations. These missed examination findings ultimately identified later aided in diagnosis.[33] Isolated abdominal pain is most frequently observed in prepubertal males, whereas postpubertal males more commonly present with testicular pain.[34] Cryptorchidism, or failed descent of the testes, can also lead to presentation of testicular torsion as abdominal pain.[35]

Ovarian and testicular torsion are both diagnoses that must be thoughtfully considered by the EM clinician because of the implications they can bear on the patient's future fertility. Timely diagnosis is imperative (**Box 2**).

Urinary tract infections and sexually transmitted infections

Numerous genitourinary infections can lead to abdominal pain. UTIs and sexually transmitted infections (STIs) can both present with dysuria, urinary frequency, urgency, and abdominal or pelvic pain. These overlapping symptoms can lead to inaccurate diagnosis and treatment. Providers tend to overdiagnose UTIs while underdiagnosing STIs.[36] Test results including urine cultures and STI testing that help differentiate these entities do not typically return during a patient's stay in the ED.

In patients with genitourinary complaints, additional systemic symptoms or abdominal or pelvic pain should broaden a clinician's differential. Associated symptoms, sexual history, and physical examination can provide additional clues to the diagnosis. In a female patient with genitourinary complaints, associated vaginal discharge or irritation decreases the likelihood of UTIs and should raise concern for STI.[37] A pelvic examination is necessary to make the clinical diagnosis of cervicitis or pelvic inflammatory disease and to determine an appropriate treatment course. In addition, the examination can identify other causes of a patient's symptoms, such as non-STIs, herpetic lesions, vaginal foreign bodies, or trauma.[38] In male patients, genitourinary

---

Box 2
Pitfalls in the diagnosis of ovarian and testicular torsion

Ovarian Torsion
- May present clinically in a similar fashion to appendicitis
- Pediatric patients, in particular, can have ovarian torsion with a normal-appearing ovary[30,32]
- A negative ultrasound does not rule out ovarian torsion[32]

Testicular Torsion
- Can present with isolated abdominal pain, particularly in prepubertal males[34]
- Perform a genitourinary examination in this population, as there typically are examination findings of testicular torsion
- Genitourinary examination can also reveal findings of cryptorchidism.

symptoms plus systemic symptoms or abdominal or pelvic pain should raise the question of prostatitis, and a digital rectal examination should be completed.[36,39] These examinations are necessary to determine appropriate antibiotics and length of treatment.

Urinalysis, which is readily available and frequently used in the ED, can demonstrate leukocyte esterase and pyuria in UTIs and STIs, including pelvic inflammatory disease and prostatitis.[36] This again highlights the importance of using other clinical clues to avoid missed diagnosis (**Box 3**).

Nephrolithiasis

Kidney stones are commonly encountered in the ED and classically present with flank pain and hematuria. There is potential to miss this diagnosis when symptoms are similar to other diagnoses or testing fails to identify nephrolithiasis. Hematuria is seen in most patients with kidney stones but can be absent in up to 33%.[40] There has been a recent review of the literature and multispecialty consensus regarding the indications for US versus CT in the workup of nephrolithiasis. This review states that CT can be avoided in younger patients (approximately 35 years old in the review) with a typical presentation of renal colic if adequate pain relief can be achieved. CT may also be avoided in middle-aged patients (approximately 55 years old in the review) if there is a prior history of nephrolithiasis. US should be used in pregnant and pediatric patients as the initial imaging study of choice. CT should be used in patients with atypical patients, older age, and persistent or uncontrolled pain (**Box 4**).[41]

Vascular

When considering missed abdominal pain diagnoses, a ruptured abdominal aortic aneurysm is one of the most feared because of its high mortality rate of 80% to 90%.[42,43] This diagnosis is missed in 42% of cases with the most common misdiagnosis being nephrolithiasis. The classic presenting symptom of abdominal pain is present in only 61% of patients, and shock and a pulsatile abdominal mass is present in less than 50%.[42] Point of care ultrasound is sensitive and specific for identifying an abdominal aortic aneurysm but typically misses retroperitoneal hemorrhage from rupture.[42,43] Still, this tool can alert the clinician to the need for expedited workup.

Acute mesenteric ischemia is a rare but frequently feared missed diagnosis in the ED. The classic teaching of "pain out of proportion to examination" has a sensitivity of about 50%. The lack of adequate screening tests adds to this diagnostic dilemma. Lactate, frequently used in the ED for evaluation of mesenteric ischemia, has sensitivities ranging from 86% to 90%, which leaves potential for missed cases (**Box 5**).[44]

Endocrine

Several systemic illnesses can present with abdominal pain, including metabolic and electrolyte derangements. Diabetic ketoacidosis (DKA) commonly presents with

---

Box 3
Ways to avoid underdiagnosing STIs in the ED

- Keep STIs on the differential when patients have genitourinary complaints
- Systemic symptoms and abdominal pain should lead to broadening of the differential
- Use physical examination findings (eg, pelvic and rectal examinations) to assess for other causes of pain and determine appropriate antibiotics and length of treatment
- Consider all possible causes of pyuria and leukocyte esterase on a urinalysis

---

Box 4
Clinical pearls for diagnosing nephrolithiasis in the ED

- Hematuria can be absent in patients with nephrolithiasis

- Ultrasound is the favored imaging modality in patients who are young with typical presentations of renal colic and well-controlled pain or in patients who are middle-aged if they have typical presentations and previous history of nephrolithiasis

- CT should be pursued if presentation is atypical for nephrolithiasis, patient is older, or pain is uncontrolled or persistent

---

abdominal pain, particularly in younger patients. This pain can be from mechanisms related to DKA itself or from underlying pathology that precipitated the DKA. More severe acidosis appears to be associated with the presence of abdominal pain.[45,46] Similarly, hypercalcemia can itself cause abdominal pain or lead to pathologies that cause pain such as constipation, peptic ulcer disease, pancreatitis, and nephrolithiasis.[47,48] Hypercalcemia is often asymptomatic until levels are greater than 12 mg/dL.[47]

Intrathoracic

Intrathoracic pathology can present with abdominal pain as the thoracic cavity is located near the abdomen. Pneumonia, pulmonary embolism, and myocardial infarction have all been noted to potentially present with abdominal pain.

Particularly in children, abdominal pain has been documented as a presenting complaint of pneumonia.[49,50] Surprisingly, the location of the pneumonia did not necessarily correlate with the presence of abdominal pain.[49] Therefore, other clinical indicators of respiratory pathology must be assessed. Certain types of respiratory infections may also have associated abdominal pain. SARS-CoV-2 (COVID-19) has been noted to cause GI symptoms. Diarrhea is most common, but abdominal pain has been noted in anywhere from less than 1% to 4% of patients.[51,52] Some patients experience isolated GI symptoms with no associated fever or respiratory symptoms.[51]

Like pneumonia, abdominal pain can be the isolated presenting symptoms of pulmonary emboli.[53] Myocardial infarction can cause abdominal pain, nausea, and vomiting, and prior studies indicate that these symptoms are more common in female patients.[54]

Malignancy

For several malignancies, the ED is the location of first presentation. Ovarian, gastric, and colon cancer can all present with abdominal pain or associated GI symptoms. Although the EM clinician might not make the diagnosis, it is important to identify the need for close follow-up as malignancies with first-time presentation to the ED are frequently more advanced and have poorer outcomes.[55,56]

Box 5
Avoiding a missed vascular diagnosis in the emergency department

- Keep abdominal aortic aneurysm and mesenteric ischemia on the differential even if patients do not have a "classic" presentation

- Use point of care ultrasound to identify the presence of abdominal aortic aneurysm and expedite CT imaging

Ovarian cancer is difficult to diagnose in early stages because of the location in the pelvis and vague-associated symptoms.[55] One study found that 20% of people diagnosed with ovarian cancer were diagnosed in the ED. Common symptoms include abdominal distention, bloating, loss of appetite, and abdominal or pelvic pain. The EM provider may also identify imaging findings concerning ovarian malignancy in an asymptomatic patient.[57]

Similar to ovarian cancer, gastric cancer is difficult to diagnose as early stages are often asymptomatic and symptoms can overlap with uncomplicated dyspepsia.[56] Common alarm symptoms include weight loss, dysphagia, upper GI bleed, anemia, and persistent vomiting, but these may be seen in other diagnoses as well. Dysphagia, weight loss, and a palpable abdominal mass are poor prognostic factors.[56]

20% to 33% of cases of colorectal cancer are initially diagnosed in the ED.[58,59] Symptoms of abdominal pain and changes in bowel habits can again be confused for other diagnoses, such as diverticular disease. CT imaging also may miss colorectal cancer.[60] Women with a history of gynecologic, irritable bowel syndrome, or diverticular disease diagnoses are at increased risk of emergency presentation of colon cancer.[59] Recent diagnosis of irritable bowel syndrome or diverticular disease is also associated with a higher rate of subsequent colon cancer diagnosis, possibly due to initial misdiagnosis.[61]

Across malignancies, lower socioeconomic groups are more likely to have emergency presentations and later stages of disease at diagnosis.[58,59,61] ED workups may be inadequate for certain GI symptoms; therefore, the ED clinician should provide instructions regarding follow-up and appropriate referrals when able, paying particular attention to resources for vulnerable populations.

DISCHARGING THE ABDOMINAL PAIN PATIENT

Many ED patients with abdominal pain do not have an established diagnosis at the time of discharge. 40% of patients younger than 50 years presenting with abdominal pain receive a nonspecific abdominal pain diagnosis upon disposition.[62] They are discharged with diagnoses such as "nausea and vomiting," "nonspecific abdominal pain," and "other gastrointestinal disorders."[1] Therefore there is some uncertainty in many cases regarding the exact cause of the patient's presenting symptoms. However, the clinician should work through the differential diagnosis to exclude life-threatening causes of abdominal pain before discharge. Despite this approach, in a study of more than 23 years of closed malpractice claims, appendicitis and "symptoms involving the abdomen and pelvis" still accounted for 1 in 20 claims. Error in diagnosis was the most common category of error attributed to ED claims. Almost half of all paid claims were attributed to a diagnostic error.[63] Abdominal pain is a chief complaint with a broad differential diagnosis, many diagnostic pitfalls, risk from a medicolegal perspective, and, most importantly, risk for the patient. The clinician must be careful, thoughtful, and methodical in the approach to discharge of the patient with abdominal pain.

Reassessment of the patient before discharge is imperative. Vital signs, discussion of the patient's level of pain and symptoms throughout the course of the evaluation, ability to tolerate oral intake, and repeat abdominal examination are essential elements of this reassessment. The clinician should address any abnormalities or concerning findings from the reassessment and document thoroughly. Cinar and colleagues[64] reported that 48% of patients at the time of discharge still reported moderate to severe pain. If the clinician discharges a patient who still reports pain, there should still be presence and documentation of normal vital signs, ability to tolerate oral intake, and a benign abdominal examination, as well as the clinician's thought process and decision making behind the discharge disposition. Discharging patients with continued discomfort can pose a risk. Patients with chronic abdominal complaints may have a concomitant acute diagnosis. Further observation of patients with continued symptoms may be warranted and needs to be determined on a case-by-case basis. In a study of appendicitis, for example, hospitals with observation units had a trend toward lower rate of missed diagnosis, lower appendiceal perforation rate, and lower abscess rate.[65]

ED clinicians should develop a consistent routine at the time of discharge to ensure that the patient's workup and treatment are complete. These steps should include reviewing discharge vital signs, assuring that all laboratory results have been reviewed and addressed, and making sure that radiographic studies have undergone a final review. This will significantly reduce risk. The breakdown of the diagnostic process leads to litigation in up to 71% of cases, with incorrect interpretation of a diagnostic test accounting for 37% of the sources of missed or delayed diagnoses.[66]

Discharge instructions should define the diagnosis, provide clear education regarding the diagnosis and any medications prescribed, give strict return precautions, and have a defined follow-up plan. If a specific diagnosis has not been definitively established, a broad diagnosis that describes the patient's presenting symptoms can be used such as "abdominal pain" or "nausea and vomiting." The broadness of the diagnosis acknowledges that there is a possibility of the presence of a more serious diagnosis. The diagnosis of "gastroenteritis" is a good example of this as that ED diagnosis commonly is seen in cases of missed appendicitis that have resulted in litigation.[66] "Constipation" is another common misdiagnosis. Return precautions should include symptoms pertinent to the patient's initial complaint that would require re-examination and may conclude with an open-ended phrase such as "or any other concerns." Follow-up planning should clearly define where the patient should follow-up and provide a specific timeline in which that visit should occur. Up to a quarter of discharged ED abdominal pain patients have a clinically relevant change in diagnosis and treatment within 30 hours.[67]

Written discharge instructions must be accompanied by verbal instructions. Patient literacy and understanding of the written discharge materials may be limited. It has been estimated that 45% to 50% of ED patients or caregivers would be unable to adequately understand their written instructions.[68] Consistent delivery of verbal instructions also assures that the provider has the opportunity to answer any questions that the patient may have. The provider should document the delivery of the verbal

---

Box 6
Steps to discharging a patient with abdominal pain without a final diagnosis

Reassess the patient before discharge
- Vital signs
- Pain level
- Ability to tolerate PO intake
- Repeat abdominal examination

Review laboratories and imaging studies to ensure they have been appropriately addressed.

Provide both written and verbal discharge instructions.
- Return precautions
- Follow-up plan

instructions.[68] Excellent communication is paramount to providing safe and effective patient care (**Box 6**).

CLINICS CARE POINTS

- When evaluating a patient with abdominal pain in the Emergency Department, use a combination of history, physical examination, and laboratory testing and imaging when appropriate for the most complete evaluation.

- Keep a broad differential for causes of a patient's abdominal pain (including GI and non-GI sources) as a less common diagnosis is unlikely to be made if it is not considered in the differential.

- Biliary pathology is one of the most frequently missed diagnoses in patients presenting with abdominal pain, so carefully evaluate patients with signs or symptoms of these diagnoses.

- Important non-GI sources of abdominal pain to consider include ovarian/testicular pathology, STIs, UTIs, nephrolithiasis, AAA, mesenteric ischemia, DKA, hypercalcemia, and pneumonia.

- In all patients, including prepubescent patients, remember that ovarian and testicular pathology can present with abdominal pain.

- When caring for patients with genitourinary complaints, keep STIs on the differential and use pelvic and rectal examinations to help guide diagnosis and treatment plans.

- When discharging a patient with abdominal pain:
  - Reassess vital signs, pain level, abdominal examination, and ability to tolerate PO intake
  - Review all laboratory and imaging results
  - Provide detailed written and verbal return precautions

REFERENCES

1. Meltzer A, Pines J, Richards L, et al. US emergency department visits for adults with abdominal and pelvic pain (2007–13): Trends in demographics, resource utilization and medication usage. Am J Emerg Med 2017;35(12):1966–9.
2. Hooker E, Mallow P, Oglesby M. Characteristics and trends of emergency department visits in the United States (2010–2014). J Emerg Med 2019;56(3):344–51.
3. Medford-Davis L, Park E, Shlamovitz G, et al. Diagnostic errors related to acute abdominal pain in the emergency department. Emerg Med J 2015;33(4):253–9.
4. Kacprzyk A, Stefura T, Chłopaś K, et al. Analysis of readmissions to the emergency department among patients presenting with abdominal pain. BMC Emerg Med 2020;20(1).
5. Soh C, Lin Z, Pan D, et al. Risk factors for emergency department unscheduled return visits. Medicina 2019;55(8):457.
6. Patterson B, Venkatesh A, AlKhawam L, et al. Abdominal computed tomography utilization and 30-day revisitation in emergency department patients presenting with abdominal pain. Acad Emerg Med 2015;22(7):803–10.
7. White D, Kaplan L, Eddy L. Characteristics of patients who return to the emergency department within 72 hours in one community hospital. Adv Emerg Nurs J 2011;33(4):344–53.
8. Ravn-Christensen C, Qvist N, Bay-Nielsen M, et al. Pathology is common in subsequent visits after admission for non-specific abdominal pain. Dan Med J 2019;66(7):A5549.

9. Osterwalder I, Özkan M, Malinovska A, et al. Acute abdominal pain: missed diagnoses, extra-abdominal conditions, and outcomes. J Clin Med 2020;9(4):899.

10. Mahajan P, Basu T, Pai C-W, et al. Factors associated with potentially missed diagnosis of appendicitis in the emergency department. JAMA Netw Open 2020;3(3):e200612.

11. Ng C, Watson C, Palmer C, et al. Evaluation of early abdominopelvic computed tomography in patients with acute abdominal pain of unknown cause: prospective randomised study. BMJ 2002;325(7377):1387.

12. Lee L, Reisner A, Binder W, et al. Repeat CT performed within one month of CT conducted in the emergency department for abdominal pain: a secondary analysis of data from a prospective multicenter study. Am J Roentgenol 2019;212(2):382–5.

13. Kabir S, Kabir S, Sun R, et al. How to diagnose an acutely inflamed appendix; a systematic review of the latest evidence. Int J Surg 2017;40:155–62.

14. Shogilev D, Duus N, Odom S, et al. Diagnosing appendicitis: evidence-based review of the diagnostic approach in 2014. West J Emerg Med 2014;15(7):859–971.

15. Sengupta A, Bax G, Paterson-Brown S. White cell count and C-reactive protein measurement in patients with possible appendicitis. Ann R Coll Surg Engl 2009;91(2):113–5.

16. Vaughn-Shaw P, Rees J, Bell E, et al. Normal inflammatory markers in appendicitis: evidence from two independent cohort studies. JRSM Short Rep 2011;(5):43.

17. Chisthi M, Surendran A, Narayanan J. RIPASA and air scoring systems are superior to alvarado scoring in acute appendicitis: diagnostic accuracy study. Ann Med Surg (Lond) 2020;59:138–42.

18. Levine C, Aizenstein O, Lehavi O, et al. Why we miss the diagnosis of appendicitis on abdominal CT: evaluation of imaging features of appendicitis incorrectly diagnosed on CT. Am J Roentgen 2005;184(3):855–9.

19. Kave M, Parooie F, Salarzaei. Pregnancy and appendicitis: a systematic review and meta-analysis on the clinical use of MRI in diagnosis of appendicitis in pregnant women. World J Emerg Surg 2019;14:37.

20. Gruber P, Silverman R, Gottesfeld S, et al. Presence of fever and leukocytosis in acute cholecystitis. Ann Emerg Med 1996;28(3):273–7.

21. Sekimoto R, Iwata K. Sensitivity of murphy's sign on the diagnosis of acute cholecystitis: is it really so insensitive. J Hepatobiliary Pancreat Sci 2019;26(10):E10.

22. Adedeji O, McAdam W. Murphy's sign, acute cholecystitis and elderly people. J R Coll Surg Edinb 1996;41(2):88–9.

23. Beliaev A, Marshall R, Booth M. C-reactive protein has a better discriminative power than white cell count in the diagnosis of acute cholecystitis. J Surg Res 2015;198(1):66–72.

24. Beliaev A, Angelo N, Booth M, et al. Evaluation of neutrophil-to-lymphocyte ratio as a potential biomarker for acute cholecystitis. J Surg Res 2017;209:93–101.

25. Padda M, Singh S, Tang S, et al. Liver test patterns with acute calculous cholecysitis and/or choledocholithiasis. Aliment Pharmacol Ther 2009;29(9):1011–8.

26. Wright G, Stillwell K, Johnson J, et al. Predicting length of stay and conversion to open cholecystectomy for acute cholecystitis using the 2013 Tokyo Guidelines in a US population. J Hepatobiliary Pancreat Sci 2015;22(11):795–801.

27. Yarmish G, Smith M, Rosen M, et al. ACR appropriateness criteria right upper quadrant pain. J Am Coll Radiol 2014;11(3):316–22.

28. Hiatt K, Ou J, Childs D. Role of ultrasound and CT in the workup of right upper quadrant pain in adults in the emergency department: a retrospective review of more than 2800 cases. Am J Roentgenol 2020;214(6):1305–10.

29. Kalimi R, Gecelter G, Caplin D, et al. Diagnosis of acute cholecystitis: sensitivity of sonography, cholecyscintigraphy, and combined sonography-cholescintigraphy. J Am Coll Surg 2001;193(6):609–13.

30. Sasaki K, Miller C. Adnexal torsion: review of the literature. J Minim Invasive Gynecol 2014;21(2):196–202.

31. McCloskey K, Grover S, Vuillermin P, et al. Ovarian torsion among girls presenting with abdominal pain: a retrospective cohort study. Emerg Med J 2012; 30(1):e11.

32. Rey-Bellet Gasser C, Gehri M, Joseph J-M, et al. Is it ovarian torsion? a systematic literature review and evaluation of prediction signs. Pediatr Emerg Care 2016; 32(4):256–61.

33. Vasconcelos-Castro S, Soares-Oliveira M. Abdominal pain in teenagers: beware of testicular torsion. J Pediatr Surg 2020;55(9):1933–5.

34. Goetz J, Roewe R, Doolittle J, et al. A comparison of clinical outcomes of acute testicular torsion between prepubertal and postpubertal males. J Pediatr Urol 2019;15(6):610–6.

35. Laher A, Ragavan S, Mehta P, et al. Testicular torsion in the emergency room: a review of detection and management strategies. Open Access Emerg Med 2020; 12:237–46.

36. Tomas ME, Getman D, Donskey CJ, et al. Overdiagnosis of urinary tract infection and underdiagnosis of sexually transmitted infection in adult women presenting to an emergency department. J Clin Microbiol 2015;53(8):2686–92.

37. Gupta K, Grigoryan L, Trautner B. Urinary tract infection. Ann Intern Med 2017; 167(7):ITC49–64.

38. Mealey K, Braverman PK, Koenigs LMP. Why a pelvic exam is needed to diagnose cervicitis and pelvic inflammatory disease. Ann Emerg Med 2019;73(4): 424–5.

39. Coker TJ, Dierfeldt DM. Acute bacterial prostatitis: diagnosis and management. Am Fam Physician 2016;93(2):114–20.

40. Kobayashi T, Nishizawa K, Mitsumori K, et al. Impact of date of onset on the absence of hematuria in patients with acute renal colic. J Urol 2003;170(4 Part 1):1093–6.

41. Moore CL, Carpenter CR, Heilbrun ML, et al. Imaging in suspected renal colic: systematic review of the literature and multispecialty consensus. J Urol 2019; 202(3):475–83.

42. Azhar B, Patel S, Holt P, et al. Misdiagnosis of ruptured abdominal aortic aneurysm: systematic review and meta-analysis. J Endovascular Ther 2014;21(4): 568–75.

43. Rubano E, Mehta N, Caputo W, et al. Systematic review: emergency department bedside ultrasonography for diagnosing suspected abdominal aortic aneurysm. Acad Emerg Med 2013;20(2):128–38.

44. Cudnik MT, Darbha S, Jones J, et al. The diagnosis of acute mesenteric ischemia: a systematic review and meta-analysis. Acad Emerg Med 2013;20(11):1087–100.

45. Campbell I. Abdominal pain in diabetic metabolic decompensation. Clinical significance. JAMA 1975;233(2):166–8.

46. Umpierrez G, Freire A. Abdominal pain in patients with hyperglycemic crises. J Crit Care 2002;17(1):63–7.

47. Carroll M, Schade D. A practical approach to hypercalcemia. Am Fam Physician 2003;67(9):1959–66.
48. Turner J. Hypercalcaemia – presentation and management. Clin Med (Lond) 2017;17(3):270–3.
49. Ravichandran D, Burge D. Pneumonia presenting with acute abdominal pain in children. Br J Surg 1996;83(12):1707–8.
50. Grief S, Loza J. Guidelines for the evaluation and treatment of pneumonia. Prim Care 2018;45(3):485–503.
51. Dorrell R, Dougherty M, Barash E, et al. Gastrointestinal and hepatic manifestations of COVID -19: a systematic review and meta-analysis. JGH Open 2020; 5(1):107–15.
52. Merola E, Armelao F, de Pretis G. Prevalence of gastrointestinal symptoms in coronavirus disease 2019 : a meta- analysis. Acta Gastroenterol Belg 2020;83: 603–15.
53. Han Y, Gong Y. Pulmonary embolism with abdominal pain as the chief complaint. Medicine 2019;98(44):e17791.
54. Herlitz J, Bang A, Karlson B, et al. Is there a gender difference in aetiology of chest pain and symptoms associated with acute myocardial infarction? Eur Jour Emerg Med 1999;6(4):311–5.
55. Ebell M, Culp M, Radke T. A systematic review of symptoms for the diagnosis of ovarian cancer. Am J Prev Med 2016;50(3):384–94.
56. Maconi G, Manes G, Porro G. Role of symptoms in diagnosis and outcome of gastric cancer. World J Gastroenterol 2008;14(8):1149.
57. Suh-Burgmann E, Alavi M. Detection of early stage ovarian cancer in a large community cohort. Cancer Med 2019;8(16):7133–40.
58. Gunnarsson H, Ekholm A, Olsson L. Emergency presentation and socioeconomic status in colon cancer. Eur J Surg Oncol 2013;39(8):831–6.
59. Renzi C, Lyratzopoulos G, Hamilton W, et al. Contrasting effects of comorbidities on emergency colon cancer diagnosis: a longitudinal data-linkage study in England. BMC Health Serv Res 2019;19(1):311.
60. Vaughan-Shaw P, Aung M, Knight H, et al. Systematic analysis of missed colorectal cancer cases and common pitfalls in diagnosis. Frontline Gastroenterol 2015;6(4):232–40.
61. Renzi C, Lyratzopoulos G, Hamilton W, et al. Opportunities for reducing emergency diagnoses of colon cancer in women and men: a data-linkage study on pre-diagnostic symptomatic presentations and benign diagnoses. Eur Jour Cancer Care 2019;28(2):e13000.
62. Day R, Fordyce J. Approach to abdominal pain. In: Cameron P, Little M, Mitra B, et al, editors. Textbook of adult emergency medicine. 5th edition. Amsterdam: Elsevier; 2020. p. 302–9.
63. Brown T, McCarthy M, Kelen G, et al. An epidemiologic study of closed emergency department malpractice claims in a national database of physician malpractice insurers. Acad Emerg Med 2010;17:553–60.
64. Cinar O, Jay L, Fosnocht D, et al. Longitudinal trends in the treatment of abdominal pain in an academic emergency department. J Emerg Med 2013;45(3): 324–31.
65. Graff L, Russell J, Seashore J, et al. False-negative and false-positive errors in abdominal pain evaluation: failure to diagnose acute appendicitis and unnecessary surgery. Acad Emerg Med 2000;7(11):1244.

66. Ferguson B, Geralds J, Petrey J, et al. Malpractice in emergency medicine – a review of risk and mitigation practices for the emergency medicine provider. J Emerg Med 2018;55(5):659–65.
67. Boendermaker A, Coolsma C, Emous M, et al. Efficacy of scheduled return visits for emergency department patients with non-specific abdominal pain. Emerg Med J 2018;35(8):499–506.
68. Taylor D, Cameron P. Discharge instructions for emergency department patients: what should we provide? J Acad Emerg Med 2000;17:86–90.

Clinical Decision Rules in the Evaluation and Management of Adult Gastrointestinal Emergencies

Kevin M. Cullison, MD*, Nathan Franck, MD

KEYWORDS

- Abdominal pain • Clinical decision rule • Appendicitis • Gastrointestinal hemorrhage

KEY POINTS

- The diagnosis and management of patients with suspected gastrointestinal emergencies is challenging as isolated history and examination findings cannot confirm or eliminate a diagnosis.
- Though several clinical decision rules have been derived and partially validated for the evaluation of suspected appendicitis, all await further validation in North America.
- There is limited evidence demonstrating the safety and efficacy of clinical decision rules for the management of upper GI bleeding in the emergency department setting.

INTRODUCTION

Abdominal pain is the most common chief complaint among patients in the emergency department (ED), accounting for over 12 million visits annually.[1] The diagnosis of many gastrointestinal (GI) emergencies can be challenging. Approximately, 1 in 6 adult patients who visit an ED for abdominal pain is admitted to the hospital or assigned a serious diagnosis.[2,3] On the contrary, the most common diagnosis among all patients in the ED with a chief complaint of abdominal pain is nonspecific abdominal pain, accounting for nearly one-third of all patients with abdominal pain.[4] Although about 80% of patients visiting the ED with abdominal pain are discharged, there is significant resource use associated with the evaluation of patients with suspected GI emergencies.[3] As detailed elsewhere in this edition of EM Clinics, most patients will undergo some form of laboratory testing with or without diagnostic imaging. The key decisions that ED providers must make for any patient with abdominal pain are whether or not to pursue abdominal imaging or to hospitalize these patients to rule-in or rule-out an acute intra-abdominal disease process. For this reason, many of the clinical decision rules

Ronald O. Perelman Department of Emergency Medicine, NYU Grossman School of Medicine, 545 1st Avenue, New York, NY 10016, USA
* Corresponding author.
E-mail address: kevin.cullison@nyulangone.org

Emerg Med Clin N Am 39 (2021) 719–732
https://doi.org/10.1016/j.emc.2021.07.001
0733-8627/21/© 2021 Elsevier Inc. All rights reserved.

(CDRs) that exist are used to develop a post-test probability for these GI emergencies so that ED physicians can make informed decisions about which patients are most likely to benefit from further testing or hospitalization. This article summarizes selected CDRs that have been developed for the management of patients with acute GI emergencies. It will also discuss important areas for future validation research as well as potential barriers to the implementation of these CDRs in the ED setting.

NEED FOR CLINICAL DECISION RULES

Before the widespread availability of computed tomography (CT) imaging, serial abdominal examinations and observation were used to help differentiate surgical from nonsurgical causes of abdominal pain in stable patients without peritoneal signs. Over the past 3 decades, there has been a dramatic increase in CT utilization for ED patients with nontraumatic abdominal pain, aimed at improving diagnostic accuracy, reducing missed diagnoses, and avoiding unnecessary hospitalizations and surgical interventions.[3,5–7] There is, however, measurable harm and cost associated with the use of CT imaging. These include prolonged ED stays, radiation exposure, as well as potential overdiagnosis and iatrogenic harm related to the discovery of incidental findings.[8–10] Although some studies have demonstrated that CT imaging significantly alters the treatment for many patients and may reduce 30-day ED return rates,[6,11] others have shown that increased rates of CT imaging are not associated with changes in the rates of diagnosis or hospitalization for many common GI emergencies, including appendicitis, gallbladder disease, and diverticulitis.[3,5] Lastly, there is evidence of practice variation among ED providers and hospitals in CT imaging and admission rates for patients with abdominal pain, and such practice variation is often cited as evidence of low-quality care.[2,12]

If properly derived and validated, CDRs could help minimize avoidable diagnostic imaging as well as hospitalizations and other interventions for patients at the lowest risk for acute GI emergencies.[13] Development of a CDR requires 3 crucial steps: (1) derivation of the rule; (2) validation of the rule in multiple different clinical settings; and (3) demonstrating that use of the CDR improves patient outcomes or reduces unnecessary resource utilization. Although many CDRs have demonstrated mixed results in terms of altering ED physician behavior or improving patient outcomes, there is evidence of decreased variation in imaging rates for patients with conditions that have well-validated CDRs such as traumatic headache or atraumatic chest pain.[14] This suggests that further research into the development of CDRs for patients with suspected GI emergencies would be beneficial. This goal was recently highlighted through a consensus conference workshop in which a panel of ED physicians selected the development of CDRs for the evaluation of nontraumatic abdominal pain to be a high priority for future research.[15]

Deriving a CDR for use in GI emergencies is challenging because patients exhibit a wide range of clinical presentations and individual history, physical examination, and laboratory findings lack sensitivity and specificity for ruling-out or ruling-in common GI emergencies such as appendicitis and cholecystitis.[16,17] Currently, there are a limited number of specific GI emergencies for which CDRs may be helpful for deciding which patients would benefit from further diagnostic testing or hospitalization. These decision rules are discussed below and relate to the diagnosis and management of acute appendicitis (AA) and GI bleeds. Because ED physicians have the most direct influence over the decision to test and hospitalize low-risk patients (as opposed to direct surgical interventions or endoscopy for high-risk patients), we will focus our discussion on the low probability cutoffs for these CDRs.

DISCUSSION

Clinical Decision Rules for the Diagnosis of Appendicitis

One of the most common abdominal surgical emergencies is AA.[18] Several CDRs have been developed to aid in the diagnosis of AA although few have undergone rigorous validation in the ED setting.[19-23] We limit our discussion here to a few simplified CDRs which have been externally validated in at least one foreign setting and show promising results. **Fig. 1** illustrates the clinical variables used to calculate the Alvarado score, the Appendicitis Inflammatory Response (AIR) score, and the Adult Appendicitis Score (AAS). **Fig. 2** summarizes the salient features of the derivation studies for these prediction rules as well as their diagnostic accuracy in validation studies at different low-probability cutoff thresholds among patients with suspected AA.

Alvarado Score

The most well-known CDR for AA, the Alvarado score, was derived in 1986 using data abstracted from the charts of 277 patients, including adults and children, admitted with suspected AA. As shown in **Fig. 1**, it consists of 8 clinical variables, many of which are used in other CDRs for AA. The Alvarado score has subsequently undergone multiple validation studies and 2 systematic reviews have summarized the performance of the Alvarado score at different cutoff thresholds.[24,25] The pooled sensitivities and specificities from these reviews are shown in **Fig. 2**. At a cutoff threshold of less than 4 or less than 5, the Alvarado score has a high sensitivity (~99%) for identifying those patients at very low risk for AA. The specificity, however, was poor at 0.17 and 0.43, respectively, because most patients without appendicitis are stratified into a moderate or high-risk category.

Using the Pauker and Kassirer threshold model of diagnosis,[26] the authors of the 2014 systematic review calculated the post-test probabilities for AA across a range of different theoretical pretest probabilities.[25] The authors assumed an acceptable AA miss rate of 3% when defining the test threshold for the low-risk group. They set a treatment threshold of 85%, which corresponds to having a negative appendectomy rate of ≤ 15%. Using the aforementioned assumptions, the authors found that a pretest probability for AA of 50% or lower and an Alvarado score less than 5 resulted in a post-test probability of less than 3%, suggesting that these patients would be appropriate for discharge or a period of observation without further testing or interventions.

Appendicitis Inflammatory Response Score

More recently, several CDRs have been derived, which incorporate the use of an inflammatory marker, C-reactive protein (CRP), into the total risk score. The AIR score (see **Fig. 1**) was developed in Sweden and includes 7 clinical variables, including CRP. Most of these variables are easy to tabulate although rebound tenderness is graded from light to strong (1, 2, or 3) and may be subject to variability depending on the experience of the physician.[21] This CDR has been validated in numerous settings across Europe and Asia.[27-30] One prospective, observational study performed in the United Kingdom (UK) calculated the AIR score on 464 consecutive patients admitted with suspected AA over a 50-week period and compared predicted outcomes to the actual management of patients by surgeons blinded to the AIR score.[28] The authors found that patients with a low probability AIR score (<5) accounted for a large proportion of admissions (48.1%) and negative appendectomies (57.1%) in the study population. The sensitivity of the AIR score at this cutoff (<5) for AA was 0.90

Clinical Variable	Alvarado Score	Appendicitis Inflammatory Response score (AIR)	Adult Appendicitis Score (AAS)
Anorexia	1		
Nausea / Vomiting	1	1	
RLQ pain		1	2
Migration of pain	1		2
RLQ tenderness	2		1 (Women age 16–49) 3 (All others)
Rebound tenderness	1	1 (Light) 2 (Medium) 3 (Strong)	
Guarding			2 (Mild) 4 (Moderate or Severe)
Fever (°C)	1 (≥37.3)	1 (≥38.5)	
Leukocytosis (x 10⁹ / L)	2 (>10.0)	1 (10.0 – 14.0) 2 (≥15.0)	1 (7.2 – 10.8) 2 (10.9 – 13.9) 3 (≥14.0)
Leftward shift (% Neutrophilia)	1 (>75%)	1 (70 – 84%) 2 (≥85%)	1 (62 – 74%) 2 (75 – 82%) 3 (≥83%)
CRP (mg/L)		1 (10 – 49) 2 (≥50)	Symptom 2 (4 – 10) Onset 3 (11 – 24) < 24 h 5 (25 – 82) 1 (≥83) / Symptom 2 (12 – 52) Onset 2 (53 – 151) > 24 h 1 (≥152)
TOTAL POSSIBLE SCORE	10	12	22

CRP = C-reactive protein; RLQ = Right Lower quadrant; Defined as Right Iliac Fossa in some studies

Fig. 1. Clinical Decision Rules for the Diagnosis of Appendicitis in Adults.

(95% confidence interval [CI], 0.84–0.95), whereas the specificity was 0.63 (95% CI, 0.58–0.68) (see **Fig. 2**). Other validation studies performed in Europe have similarly demonstrated that a low-risk AIR score has a superior specificity in comparison to the Alvarado score, allowing more patients to be stratified as low-risk and potentially safe for discharge from the ED without imaging.[27–29]

A pre-post interventional study performed across 21 different hospitals in Sweden compared the outcomes of patients with suspected AA before and after implementation of the AIR score algorithm.[30] Importantly, AIR scores were recorded by ED physicians who were advised to consider outpatient observation for patients with a low-risk score of less than 5. The primary outcome was the proportion of negative appendectomies and secondary outcomes included the rate of admissions, missed diagnoses, and imaging studies performed. Implementation of the AIR score resulted in fewer negative appendectomies (1.6 vs 3.2%, P = .030), fewer admissions (29.5 vs 42.8%, P<.001), and less imaging (19.2 vs 34.5%, P<.001) among the low-risk patient cohort. There was no difference in the rate of missed AA among low-risk patients in the preintervention and postintervention cohorts. The authors concluded that use of the AIR score can safely reduce the need for diagnostic imaging among patients with a low-risk score (<5). Further study is needed to validate the use of the AIR score in other settings including in North America.

Adult Appendicitis Score

The AAS was derived in Finland and, like the AIR score, also consists of 7 clinical variables.[22] There are, however, several differences as illustrated in **Fig. 1**. Patients are assigned points based on the presence of guarding (instead of rebound) and laboratory markers, including WBC count, percent neutrophilia, and CRP levels are stratified into a larger number of subgroups, with CRP being further stratified depending on whether symptomatology has been ongoing for more or less than 24 hours. Furthermore, women of reproductive age (16–49 years) were assigned 1 point for RLQ tenderness instead of 3 points because of the higher rate of negative appendectomies observed among this demographic in prior studies.[31]

		Alvarado Score	Appendicitis Inflammatory Response Score (AIR)	Adult Appendicitis Score (AAS)
Derivation Studies				
Study Type		Retrospective, single-center	Prospective, multi-center	Prospective, single-center
Location		U.S.A.	Sweden	Finland
N		305	316	725
Inclusion		Patients (ages 4–80 yr) hospitalized with suspected AA	Patients (all ages) hospitalized with suspected AA	Patients (age ≥16) hospitalized with suspected AA
Primary Outcome		Surgically confirmed AA	Histopathologic confirmation	Histopathologic confirmation
Follow-up		Duration of hospital stay	1 month medical record review	2 week medical record review
SN [95% CI] SP [95% CI]		<5: 0.97 [0.94 – 0.98][a] 0.38 [0.28 – 0.46]	<5: 0.96 [0.89 – 0.99][b] 0.73 [0.70 – 0.75]	<11: 0.96 [0.93 – 0.98][c] 0.54 [0.52 – 0.56]
Validation Studies				
Low Probability Cutoff	SN [95% CI] SP [95% CI]	<4: 0.99 [0.91 – 1.00][d] 0.17 [0.06 – 0.42] <5: 0.99 [0.97 – 0.99][e] 0.43 [0.36 – 0.51]	<5: 0.90 [0.84 – 0.95][f] 0.63 [0.58 – 0.68]	<11: 0.95 [0.92 – 0.96][g] 0.60 [0.58 – 0.62]
Optimal Low Probability Cutoff for Men[h]	SP [95% CI] Failure Rate	<2: 0.06 [0.05 – 0.06] 0.0%	<3: 0.25 [0.24 – 0.25] 2.4%	<7: 0.21 [0.20 – 0.21] 5.0%
Optimal Low Probability Cutoff for Women[h]	SP [95% CI] Failure Rate	<4: 0.41 [0.40 – 0.41] 3.7%	<4: 0.52 [0.51 – 0.52] 3.5%	<9: 0.63 [0.63 – 0.64] 3.7%

Acute Appendicitis = AA; Sensitivity = SN; Specificity = SP; Failure Rate = False Negatives / (True Negatives + False Negatives)
References:
[a] Data from Alvarado. 1986   [d] Data from Ebell MH, Shinholser J. 2014 (systematic review)   [g] Data from Sammalkorpi et al. 2017
[b] Data from Andersson M, Andersson RE. 2008   [e] Data from Ohle et al. 2011 (systematic review)   [h] Data from Bhangu et al. 2020
[c] Data from Sammalkorpi et al. 2014   [f] Data from Scott et al. 2015

Fig. 2. Comparison of Derivation Studies and Diagnostic Accuracy of Clinical Decision Rules for Appendicitis in Adults.

A prospective validation study performed on the AAS score at 2 hospitals in Finland from 2014 to 2015 enrolled 908 adult patients with suspected AA.[32] Adult patients with a low-risk score (<11) were advised to be discharged without imaging. Importantly, physicians were permitted to deviate from the AAS recommendations and could perform or forgo imaging or other interventions at their own discretion. In comparison to data from the original derivation study, the use of the AAS score helped to reduce the negative appendectomy rate from 18.2% to 8.2% (P<.0001) among all patients with suspected appendicitis although there was also an observed doubling of the pre-operative imaging rates from 20.9% to 40.1% among all patients. The AAS score had a high sensitivity of 0.95 (95% CI, 0.92–0.96) among patients with a low-risk score (<11) although 7.4% patients (23 of 309) in the low-risk cohort had AA (see **Fig. 2**). It is worth noting that many physicians did not adhere to the recommendations of the AAS score as 51.5% of patients in the low-risk cohort underwent imaging before discharge. The authors concluded that the AAS score is a reliable risk stratification tool for reducing negative appendectomy rates without mandatory imaging among all patients with suspected AA. This CDR also awaits further validation studies in other ED settings.

The Validation of Gender-Specific Low-Risk Cutoff Scores for Appendicitis

Recently, a large multicenter prospective trial across 154 hospitals in the UK compared the diagnostic accuracy of 15 different CDRs for the diagnosis of AA.[33] In this study, 5345 consecutive adult patients, ages 16 to 45 years, admitted to the hospital with suspected AA were enrolled. Clinical history, examination findings, and laboratory and imaging results were prospectively collected and outcomes were tracked for 30 days after the initial presentation. The authors sought to identify the CDR, which yields the highest specificity among patients classified as low-risk for AA while maintaining a low failure rate (false negatives/[false negatives + true negatives]) of less than 5%. The desire to minimize the failure rate among low-risk patients resulted in lower optimal cut-off thresholds than what were proposed in the initial derivation studies for each CDR. Because of the higher rates of negative appendectomies among women in the UK and distinct differential diagnoses that exist among men and women with right lower quadrant pain, the authors preplanned to stratify the validation of the CDRs by gender. The authors observed significantly higher rates of negative appendectomies in women versus men (28.2 vs 12.1%) in this study. They found that an AAS score achieved the highest specificity (63.1%) among female patients without AA while maintaining a failure rate of 3.7% when using a cutoff score of less than 9. Among men, the AIR score was the optimal model, achieving a specificity of 24.7% and a failure rate of 2.4% using a cut-off score of less than 3. Both the AAS and the AIR scores were able to correctly stratify a larger proportion of patients without AA into the low-risk category (or achieve greater specificity) than the Alvarado score (see **Fig. 2**).

Caveats and Bottom Line: Clinical Decision Rules for Adults with Suspected Appendicitis

It should be noted that many of the newer CDRs for AA were derived in Europe where the management approach to patients with suspected AA may differ from practices in the United States. In a few of the UK validation studies described earlier,[28,33] imaging studies (CT or ultrasonography) were performed on less than 70% of patients, whereas preoperative imaging rates in the United States among adults with suspected AA typically exceeds 80% and CT is preferentially performed over ultrasound.[34,35] This fact combined with the higher negative appendectomy rates reported in some European countries compared with the United States suggests there are likely distinct test and treatment thresholds among ED physicians and surgeons in different international settings. Moreover, in the aforementioned systematic review by Ebell, the authors assumed an acceptable missed diagnosis rate of 3%.[25] Prior surveys of ED physicians exploring acceptable miss rates for acute myocardial infarction suggest that many physicians may not tolerate a miss rate above 1%.[36] Decreasing the acceptable missed diagnosis rate below 3% would further lower the test threshold and allow fewer patients to forgo further testing and imaging. Ultimately, the risks of a missed diagnosis or a negative appendectomy will vary according to a patient's estimated pretest probability for a disease so physicians must weigh these potential risks against the potential benefits and harms of CT imaging carefully when deciding which patients are most likely to benefit from further testing.

In most of the aforementioned derivation and validation studies, the patient population was limited to inpatients with suspected AA and physical examinations were often performed by members of the surgical team. These facts may limit the generalizability of these CDRs among all undifferentiated ED patients with abdominal pain.

Although each of the CDRs discussed earlier has a high sensitivity for ruling out AA among patients with a low probability score, impact studies performed to date have shown either modest or no benefit to the use of these CDRs over clinical gestalt.[30,37,38] None of the CDRs discussed have been endorsed for use by any emergency medicine professional societies. Until these CDRs are shown to improve patient outcomes or safely reduce health care resource utilization in a variety of settings, they are not appropriate for widespread adoption into clinical practice. Because many ED physicians may be reluctant to accept even a low missed diagnosis rate among patients with low-probability risk scores, the future development and validation of shared decision-making tools for patients at low-risk for AA may be helpful for implementing these CDRs into practice.

CLINICAL DECISION RULES FOR THE MANAGEMENT OF UPPER GASTROINTESTINAL BLEEDING

Upper gastrointestinal bleeding (UGIB) is a common ED presentation and approximately 67 per 100,000 adults are hospitalized each year with a UGIB.[39] Because the severity of a UGIB can vary widely, ED physicians must routinely use history, physical examination, and laboratory findings to determine appropriate patient disposition. To guide management and to assess the severity of UGIB, multiple CDRs have been developed. Some of these CDRs require endoscopic findings to be calculated, which greatly limits any potential applicability in an undifferentiated ED population. Several rules, however, do not require endoscopic findings including the AIMS65 rule, the Glasgow-Blatchford Bleeding Score (GBS), and the Rockall Score for Upper GI Bleeding (Pre-Endoscopy) making them potentially useful in the ED.

Rockall Score for Upper Gastrointestinal Bleeding (Pre-endoscopy)

The Rockall score is designed to determine mortality in patients with UGIB based on risk factors before (clinical Rockall) and after endoscopy (complete score) (**Fig. 3**A). As the scope of this analysis is ED-focused, the complete score will not be discussed as endoscopy data are typically unavailable. This score was developed prospectively by analyzing 4185 cases of UGIB across 74 hospitals in the UK. The score consists of 3 clinical variables, which assign different point values based on a patient's age, comorbidities, and the presence of shock. This score was validated on a second cohort of 1625 patients. The score showed a strong correlation with mortality in both the derivation and validation cohorts. A score of 0 demonstrated a sensitivity of 0.99 (95%, 0.99–1.00) and a specificity of 0.17 (95% CI, 0.17–0.17) for predicting survival (**Fig. 4**).[40]

Although the clinical Rockall score is easy to calculate and includes the clinically relevant outcome of mortality, its utility in the ED setting is limited as the pre-endoscopic Rockall score was not shown to be predictive of other patient-centric outcomes such as the risk of rebleeding or the need for a hospital intervention. Moreover, the comorbidity variable is broadly defined. Patients can be assigned a score of "2" for having any of 21 comorbid conditions that may be difficult to remember.

Glasgow-Blatchford Bleeding Score

The GBS is designed to predict which UGIB patients will need a clinical intervention. This composite outcome included receiving a transfusion, endoscopic or operative intervention, death, or evidence of rebleeding. These clinical interventions were used as a surrogate outcome to determine who needs admission as it was assumed that patients not meeting these criteria do not need or benefit from hospitalization. The score was derived using a retrospective data set of 1748 admitted patients with UGIB across 19 hospitals in Scotland and validated internally on 197 prospectively enrolled patients admitted in 3 hospitals in Scotland. The score ranges from 0 to 23 and is calculated from 7 clinical variables including elements from the clinical history, examination, and laboratory findings (**Fig. 3**B). In the derivation and validation data sets, patients with a score of 0 had a 0.3% and 0.5% need for intervention, respectively. In the derivation group, a GBS score of 0 had a sensitivity of 0.99 (95% CI, 0.98–1.00) and a specificity of 0.28 (95% CI, 0.27–0.29) for identifying patients who will not need an intervention (see **Fig. 4**). The authors concluded that the GBS score could determine which patients with UGIB are safe for outpatient management.[41]

Strengths of this score include the use of clinically relevant outcomes and its ease of use. Weaknesses of this CDR are that it was derived from patients hospitalized for UGIB rather than all comers to the ED, and the CDR also does not consider longer-term outcomes beyond the index admission.

AIMS65

AIMS65 is another CDR designed to predict mortality for patients with UGIB. It was derived and validated using a large administrative database of inpatients from 187 US hospitals. Patients with UGIB were identified for inclusion using discharge diagnosis codes. The primary outcome was mortality during the index hospitalization. The score ranges from 0 to 5 and is calculated from 5 clinical variables, which are summarized by the acronym AIMS65 (**Fig. 3**C). The AIMS65 score was shown to have a strong positive correlation with mortality in the initial derivation and validation cohorts. In the validation cohort, a score of 0 had a sensitivity of 0.98 (95% CI, 0.96–0.99) and specificity of 0.20 (95% CI, 0.20–0.20) for predicting survival to hospital discharge (see **Fig. 4**).[42]

The primary advantages of the AIMS65 CDR are its ease of calculation and its reliance on a limited number of clinical variables that are readily available in the ED. Limitations of this score are that it was derived from a retrospective database of hospitalized patients using diagnostic billing codes rather than undifferentiated ED patients with UGIB, and similar to the GBS score, it did not consider outcomes beyond the index hospital admission.

The Validation of Clinical Decision Rules for Upper Gastrointestinal Bleeding

There are multiple validation studies that directly compare the ability of these CDRs to predict 30-day adverse events. One systematic review compared the predictive value of these CDRs for serious adverse events defined as a composite of death, recurrent UGIB, or need for intervention within 30 days of index visit. Using pooled data, a low-risk GBS cutoff score of 0 had a greater sensitivity although lower specificity for predicting adverse 30-day outcomes, compared to low-risk Rockall and AIMS65 scores (see **Fig. 4**).[43]

Reinforcing these findings, a multicenter, international ED-based study examined the performance of these 3 scores for predicting the composite outcome of transfusion, endoscopic or interventional radiology treatment, surgery, or 30-day mortality.

A

Clinical Variable		Points
Age	<60	0
	60 – 79	1
	≥80	2
Shock	SBP≥100 and HR<100	0
	SBP≥100 and HR≥100	1
	SBP<100	2
Comorbidities	None	0
	Comorbidities (except for renal failure, liver failure, and/or disseminated malignancy)	2
	Renal failure, liver failure, and/or disseminated malignancy	3
TOTAL POSSIBLE SCORE		7

B

Clinical Variable		Points
BUN (mg/dL)	<18.2	0
	18.2 –22.3	2
	22.4 – 28	3
	28 – 70	4
	>70	6
Hemoglobin (g/dL)	>13 (men) or >12 (women)	0
	12-13 (men) or 10 – 12 (women)	1
	10 – 12 (men)	3
	<10 (men or women)	6
Systolic Blood Pressure	>110	0
	100 – 109	1
	90 – 99	2
	<90	3
	HR ≥100	1
	Melena	1
	Syncope	2
	Liver disease	2
	Cardiac failure	2
TOTAL POSSIBLE SCORE		23

C

Clinical Variable	Points
Albumin<3 g/dL	1
INR>1.5	1
Altered Mental Status	1
SBP ≤ 90	1
Age ≥ 65	1
TOTAL POSSIBLE SCORE	5

Fig. 3. Clinical decision scores for upper gastrointestinal bleeding. (*A*) Clinical Rockall Score (Pre-Endoscopy). (*B*) Glasgow-Blatchford Bleeding Score. (*C*) AIMS65 Score. BUN, blood urea nitrogen; HR, heart rate (beats per minute); INR, international normalized ratio; SBP, systolic blood pressure.

		Clinical Rockall Score	Glasgow-Blatchford Bleeding Score	AIMS65
Derivation Studies				
Study Type		Prospective, multicenter	Retrospective, multicenter	Retrospective, multicenter
Location		England	Scotland	U.S.A.
N		4,185	1,748	29,222
Inclusion		Patients with UGIB identified in the ED, operating room, endoscopy unit, or wards	Patients (age ≥ 15) admitted with UGIB	Patients (age ≥ 18) with a 1° discharge diagnosis of UGIB from an inpatient claims database
Primary Outcome		Mortality	Composite (transfusion, endoscopic or operative intervention, evidence of rebleeding, or death)	Mortality
Follow-up		Duration of hospital stay	Duration of hospital stay	Duration of hospital stay
Low Probability Cutoff	SN [95% CI]	<1: 0.99 [0.99 – 1.00][a]	<1: 0.99 [0.98-1.00][b]	<1: 0.98 [0.96 – 0.99][c]
	SP [95% CI]	0.17 [0.17 – 0.17]	0.28 [0.27-0.29]	0.20 [0.20 – 0.20]
Validation Studies				
Low Probability Cutoff[d]	SN [95% CI]	<1: 0.93 [0.91-0.94]	<1: 0.99 [0.98-1.00]	<1: 0.78 [0.73-0.83]
	SP [95% CI]	0.38 [0.18-0.20]	0.08 [0.07-0.09]	0.49 [0.45-0.53]

Sensitivity = SN, Specificity = SP, Upper Gastrointestinal Bleeding = UGIB, Emergency Department = ED

References:
[a] Data from Rockall 1996   [d] Data from Saltzman 2011
[b] Data from Blatchford 2000   [e] Data from Ramaekers 2016

Fig. 4. Comparison of derivation studies and diagnostic accuracy of clinical decision rules for upper GI bleeds.

A GBS score of ≤1 had a higher sensitivity (98.6%) for identifying patients at low-risk for adverse 30-day outcomes compared to AIMS65 and clinical Rockall scores of 0 which had sensitivities of 81.6% and 95.6%, respectively. Importantly, there was also a lower failure rate (false negative/[false negative + true negative]) among patients with a low-risk GBS score of ≤1 as only 3.4% of these patients required an intervention or died within 30 days compared with 14% and 25% of patients with low-risk Rockall and AIMS65 scores, respectively.[44] Multiple other retrospective and prospective validation studies demonstrated similar results when examining outcome measures of mortality, need for transfusion, and interventions.[45–48] Although there are many head-to-head comparisons of these CDRs as discussed earlier, there are still no large, prospective studies comparing the performance of these CDRs to clinical gestalt or contemporary practice.

Using Clinical Decision Rules for Upper Gastrointestinal Bleeding to Reduce Hospital Admissions

A few pre-post intervention studies have attempted to demonstrate the safety of the GBS score for identifying patients who can be safely managed in the outpatient setting. One such study in the UK first prospectively validated the GBS score in an observational cohort and discovered that the diagnostic accuracy of this CDR varied with age. They therefore modified the inclusion criteria for the intervention part of the trial such that only patients with a GBS ≤2 and age less than 70 years were deemed low-risk and safe for outpatient management. Notably, enrolled patients were also scheduled for outpatient endoscopy the following weekday morning. In the postintervention cohort, 304 patients were enrolled and 104 (34.2%) had a score of ≤ 2 and age less than 70 years. Only 30.7% of these patients (32 of 104) were managed as an outpatient with all but one patient receiving endoscopy. The reason some low-risk patients were admitted to the hospital varied and included the presence of a significant comorbidity, time of day, alcohol intoxication, and lacking a person to accompany the patient to home. None of the 104 patients deemed low-risk, whether managed as an inpatient or outpatient required endoscopic therapy, transfusion, surgery, or died. These findings provide evidence that there may be a low-risk cohort of patients with UGIB that could be safely managed in the outpatient setting. This study was not very pragmatic, however, as it may not be feasible for most hospitals to guarantee rapid outpatient endoscopy on the following weekday.[49]

Another pre-post intervention study used a more conservative GBS score of 0 to classify patients as low-risk. In the preintervention cohort, only 6% of low-risk patients (3 of 53) were not admitted to the hospital. In the postintervention cohort, 123 of 491 (22%) with UGIB were classified as low-risk and 68% (84 of 123) were managed as outpatients. All these patients were offered outpatient endoscopy but only 40% underwent it. None of the patients classified as low-risk needed intervention or died.[50]

Both the aforementioned studies suggest that the GBS score might be useful for identifying low-risk patients with UGIB that can be safely managed in the outpatient setting although these studies included strict inclusion criteria so further pragmatic studies in North America are still needed.

Caveats and Bottom Line: Clinical Decision Rules for Upper Gastrointestinal Bleeding

CDRs for UGIB are a potentially useful tool for identifying patients who can be safely managed in the outpatient setting. These CDRs offer the ability to risk stratify patients with UGIB without endoscopy results and may predict 30-day adverse events including mortality and the need for intervention. As discussed earlier, the GBS score has a higher sensitivity for identifying patients at low-risk for adverse events compared with the clinical Rockall and AIMS65 scores. It should be noted that the lack of an intervention (transfusion, endoscopic intervention, or surgery) while hospitalized is a surrogate outcome for safe hospital discharge and may not account for other potential benefits of inpatient admission such as the administration of intravenous proton pump inhibitors which may not be easily replicated in an outpatient setting. Lastly, prior studies suggesting the potential safety of discharging patients with a low-risk GBS score are not easily generalizable as most of these studies arranged next-day outpatient endoscopy and many patients were admitted despite being deemed low-risk by the CDR.

There are currently no widely recognized national practice guidelines from professional organizations that support the use of these CDRs in determining which patients with a UGIB can be safely managed as an outpatient. Further prospective randomized studies comparing use of these CDRs to contemporary practice are needed.

SUMMARY

Evaluating ED patients with abdominal pain and suspected GI emergencies is a challenging task. The routine use of advanced imaging or hospitalization of patients with suspected GI emergencies may reduce the incidence of missed diagnoses but at the cost of significant health care resources without clear benefit and even potential harm for those patients at low-risk for acute disease or adverse outcomes. Further validation of CDRs for ED patients with suspected GI emergencies is warranted as preliminary work shows these tools may be helpful for identifying patients at low-risk for AA or dangerous UGIB. Before these CDRs are implemented, additional trials are needed to confirm that these CDRs improve on current practice. Although we limited our discussion to simplified CDRs that can be easily calculated in the ED, advancements in electronic health record technology may permit the use of more complex clinical decision support tools in the future that can take into consideration local disease epidemiology and more complex clinical variables. Importantly, no CDR is meant to entirely supersede clinical judgment but should instead be used to augment and inform clinical decision-making by quantifying a patient's risk for disease. When properly validated, CDRs can serve as a simplified and objective tool for risk stratifying patients and may lessen the cognitive burden of decision-making, particularly for more junior clinicians facing diagnostic uncertainty in a hectic work environment. As various physician and patient-level factors, including lack of comfort with a missed diagnosis or inability to secure proper outpatient follow-up, may serve as barriers to the future adoption of these CDRs into practice, future research should be directed toward the development of shared decision-making tools for low-risk patients.

DISCLOSURE

The authors have nothing to disclose.

REFERENCES

1. Rui P, Kang K. National Hospital Ambulatory Medical Care Survey: 2017 emergency department summary tables. National Center for Health Statistics. Available at: https://www.cdc.gov/nchs/data/nhamcs/web_tables/2017_ed_web_tables-508.pdf.
2. Khojah I, Li S, Luo Q, et al. The relative contribution of provider and ED-level factors to variation among the top 15 reasons for ED admission. Am J Emerg Med 2017;35(9):1291–7.
3. Bhuiya FPS, McCaig LF. Emergency department visits for chest pain and abdominal pain: United States, 1999-2008. Hyattsville, MD: National Center for Health Statistics; 2010.
4. Cervellin G, Mora R, Ticinesi A, et al. Epidemiology and outcomes of acute abdominal pain in a large urban Emergency Department: retrospective analysis of 5,340 cases. Ann Transl Med 2016;4(19):362.
5. Pines JM. Trends in the rates of radiography use and important diagnoses in emergency department patients with abdominal pain. Med Care 2009;47(7):782–6.
6. Patterson BW, Venkatesh AK, AlKhawam L, et al. Abdominal Computed Tomography Utilization and 30-day Revisitation in Emergency Department Patients Presenting With Abdominal Pain. Acad Emerg Med 2015;22(7):803–10.
7. Krajewski S, Brown J, Phang PT, et al. Impact of computed tomography of the abdomen on clinical outcomes in patients with acute right lower quadrant pain: a meta-analysis. Can J Surg 2011;54(1):43–53.
8. Rogers W, Hoffman J, Noori N. Harms of CT scanning prior to surgery for suspected appendicitis. Evid Based Med 2015;20(1):3–4.
9. Kocher KE, Meurer WJ, Desmond JS, et al. Effect of testing and treatment on emergency department length of stay using a national database. Acad Emerg Med 2012;19(5):525–34.
10. Morgan AE, Berland LL, Ananyev SS, et al. Extraurinary Incidental Findings on CT for Hematuria: The Radiologist's Role and Downstream Cost Analysis. AJR Am J Roentgenol 2015;204(6):1160–7.
11. Rosen MP, Siewert B, Sands DZ, et al. Value of abdominal CT in the emergency department for patients with abdominal pain. Eur Radiol 2003;13(2):418–24.
12. Levine MB, Moore AB, Franck C, et al. Variation in use of all types of computed tomography by emergency physicians. Am J Emerg Med 2013;31(10):1437–42.
13. McGinn TG, Guyatt GH, Wyer PC, et al. Users' guides to the medical literature: XXII: how to use articles about clinical decision rules. Evidence-Based Medicine Working Group. JAMA 2000;284(1):79–84.

14. Taylor RA, Melnick E, Fleishman W, et al. The Impact of Risk Standardization on Variation in CT Use and Emergency Physician Profiling. AJR Am J Roentgenol 2018;211(2):392–9.
15. Gunn ML, Marin JR, Mills AM, et al. A report on the Academic Emergency Medicine 2015 consensus conference "Diagnostic imaging in the emergency department: a research agenda to optimize utilization". Emerg Radiol 2016;23(4): 383–96.
16. Benabbas R, Hanna M, Shah J, et al. Diagnostic Accuracy of History, Physical Examination, Laboratory Tests, and Point-of-care Ultrasound for Pediatric Acute Appendicitis in the Emergency Department: A Systematic Review and Meta-analysis. Acad Emerg Med 2017;24(5):523–51.
17. Jain A, Mehta N, Secko M, et al. History, Physical Examination, Laboratory Testing, and Emergency Department Ultrasonography for the Diagnosis of Acute Cholecystitis. Acad Emerg Med 2017;24(3):281–97.
18. Coward S, Kareemi H, Clement F, et al. Incidence of Appendicitis over Time: A Comparative Analysis of an Administrative Healthcare Database and a Pathology-Proven Appendicitis Registry. PLoS One. 2016;11(11):e0165161.
19. Alvarado A. A practical score for the early diagnosis of acute appendicitis. Ann Emerg Med 1986;15(5):557–64.
20. Chong CF, Adi MI, Thien A, et al. Development of the RIPASA score: a new appendicitis scoring system for the diagnosis of acute appendicitis. Singapore Med J 2010;51(3):220–5.
21. Andersson M, Andersson RE. The appendicitis inflammatory response score: a tool for the diagnosis of acute appendicitis that outperforms the Alvarado score. World J Surg 2008;32(8):1843–9.
22. Sammalkorpi HE, Mentula P, Leppaniemi A. A new adult appendicitis score improves diagnostic accuracy of acute appendicitis–a prospective study. BMC Gastroenterol 2014;14:114.
23. Mikaere H, Zeng I, Lauti M, et al. Derivation and validation of the APPEND score: an acute appendicitis clinical prediction rule. ANZ J Surg 2018;88(4):E303–7.
24. Ohle R, O'Reilly F, O'Brien KK, et al. The Alvarado score for predicting acute appendicitis: a systematic review. BMC Med 2011;9:139.
25. Ebell MH, Shinholser J. What are the most clinically useful cutoffs for the Alvarado and Pediatric Appendicitis Scores? A systematic review. Ann Emerg Med 2014; 64(4):365–372 e2.
26. Pauker SG, Kassirer JP. The threshold approach to clinical decision making. N Engl J Med 1980;302(20):1109–17.
27. Kollar D, McCartan DP, Bourke M, et al. Predicting acute appendicitis? A comparison of the Alvarado score, the Appendicitis Inflammatory Response Score and clinical assessment. World J Surg 2015;39(1):104–9.
28. Scott AJ, Mason SE, Arunakirinathan M, et al. Risk stratification by the Appendicitis Inflammatory Response score to guide decision-making in patients with suspected appendicitis. Br J Surg 2015;102(5):563–72.
29. de Castro SM, Unlu C, Steller EP, et al. Evaluation of the appendicitis inflammatory response score for patients with acute appendicitis. World J Surg 2012; 36(7):1540–5.
30. Andersson M, Kolodziej B, Andersson RE, et al. Randomized clinical trial of Appendicitis Inflammatory Response score-based management of patients with suspected appendicitis. Br J Surg 2017;104(11):1451–61.
31. Seetahal SA, Bolorunduro OB, Sookdeo TC, et al. Negative appendectomy: a 10-year review of a nationally representative sample. Am J Surg 2011;201(4):433–7.

32. Sammalkorpi HE, Mentula P, Savolainen H, et al. The Introduction of Adult Appendicitis Score Reduced Negative Appendectomy Rate. Scand J Surg 2017;106(3): 196–201.
33. Bhangu A, Collaborative RSGobotWMR. Evaluation of appendicitis risk prediction models in adults with suspected appendicitis. Br J Surg 2020;107(1):73–86.
34. Collaborative S, Cuschieri J, Florence M, et al. Negative appendectomy and imaging accuracy in the Washington State Surgical Care and Outcomes Assessment Program. Ann Surg 2008;248(4):557–63.
35. Wang RC, Kornblith AE, Grupp-Phelan J, et al. Trends in Use of Diagnostic Imaging for Abdominal Pain in U.S. Emergency Departments. AJR Am J Roentgenol 2021;216(1):200–8.
36. Schriger DL, Menchine M, Wiechmann W, et al. Emergency Physician Risk Estimates and Admission Decisions for Chest Pain: A Web-Based Scenario Study. Ann Emerg Med 2018;72(5):511–22.
37. Tan WJ, Acharyya S, Chew MH, et al. Randomized control trial comparing an Alvarado Score-based management algorithm and current best practice in the evaluation of suspected appendicitis. World J Emerg Surg 2020;15(1):30.
38. Golden SK, Harringa JB, Pickhardt PJ, et al. Prospective evaluation of the ability of clinical scoring systems and physician-determined likelihood of appendicitis to obviate the need for CT. Emerg Med J 2016;33(7):458–64.
39. Wuerth BA, Rockey DC. Changing Epidemiology of Upper Gastrointestinal Hemorrhage in the Last Decade: A Nationwide Analysis. Dig Dis Sci 2018;63(5): 1286–93.
40. Rockall TA, Logan RF, Devlin HB, et al. Risk assessment after acute upper gastrointestinal haemorrhage. Gut. 1996;38(3):316–21.
41. Blatchford O, Murray WR, Blatchford M. A risk score to predict need for treatment for upper-gastrointestinal haemorrhage. Lancet. 2000;356(9238):1318–21.
42. Saltzman JR, Tabak YP, Hyett BH, et al. A simple risk score accurately predicts in-hospital mortality, length of stay, and cost in acute upper GI bleeding. Gastrointest Endosc 2011;74(6):1215–24.
43. Ramaekers R, Mukarram M, Smith CA, et al. The Predictive Value of Preendoscopic Risk Scores to Predict Adverse Outcomes in Emergency Department Patients With Upper Gastrointestinal Bleeding: A Systematic Review. Acad Emerg Med 2016;23(11):1218–27.
44. Stanley AJ, Laine L, Dalton HR, et al. Comparison of risk scoring systems for patients presenting with upper gastrointestinal bleeding: international multicentre prospective study. BMJ 2017;356:i6432.
45. Chen IC, Hung MS, Chiu TF, et al. Risk scoring systems to predict need for clinical intervention for patients with nonvariceal upper gastrointestinal tract bleeding. Am J Emerg Med 2007;25(7):774–9.
46. Chandra S, Hess EP, Agarwal D, et al. External validation of the Glasgow-Blatchford Bleeding Score and the Rockall Score in the US setting. Am J Emerg Med 2012;30(5):673–9.
47. Yaka E, Yilmaz S, Dogan NO, et al. Comparison of the Glasgow-Blatchford and AIMS65 scoring systems for risk stratification in upper gastrointestinal bleeding in the emergency department. Acad Emerg Med 2015;22(1):22–30.
48. Schiefer M, Aquarius M, Leffers P, et al. Predictive validity of the Glasgow Blatchford Bleeding Score in an unselected emergency department population in continental Europe. Eur J Gastroenterol Hepatol 2012;24(4):382–7.

49. Stephens JR, Hare NC, Warshow U, et al. Management of minor upper gastrointestinal haemorrhage in the community using the Glasgow Blatchford Score. Eur J Gastroenterol Hepatol 2009;21(12):1340–6.
50. Stanley AJ, Ashley D, Dalton HR, et al. Outpatient management of patients with low-risk upper-gastrointestinal haemorrhage: multicentre validation and prospective evaluation. Lancet. 2009;373(9657):42–7.

Laboratory Tests in the Patient with Abdominal Pain

Sreeja Natesan, MD[a],*, Elizabeth Barrall Werley, MD[b]

KEYWORDS

• Abdominal pain • Laboratory • Diagnostic • Testing • Emergency department

KEY POINTS

• Workup of abdominal pain should begin with a detailed history and physical exam, augmented by laboratory and imaging studies to narrow the differential.
• Caution should be taken regarding the over-reliance on testing, including laboratory studies, in the workup of abdominal pain.
• Laboratory results should always be reviewed in context to the clinical presentation.
• Anticipatory guidance and a plan for further workup with primary care or specialist follow-up should be provided for inconclusive or non-diagnostic encounters.

INTRODUCTION

Abdominal pain is one of the most common complaints seen in emergency departments (ED).[1,2] In 2017, according to the National Hospital Ambulatory Medical Care Survey, "stomach and abdominal pain, cramps, and spasms" were the leading cause of ED visits across all patients.[3] Vomiting was also noted to be in the top ten complaints at presentation.[3] Abdominal pain complaints have been increasing over time, as demonstrated from 1999 to 2008, in which the complaints of abdominal pain unrelated to injury increased 31.8% in adult patients presenting to the ED.[4] There has also been an increase in resource utilization, as arrival by ambulance increased by 26.9% over a similar timeframe, and the use of advanced imaging rose by 122.6%.[4] Despite this increase in ED presentations, there was no trend in terms of being triaged at a higher level of acuity, of having findings that resulted in a significant or potentially dangerous diagnosis, or visits that necessitated admission, required transfer to another facility, or resulted in death.[4]

This leaves the emergency physician in a diagnostic dilemma as the differential diagnosis for abdominal pain and other gastrointestinal (GI) symptoms can be vast.

[a] Division of Emergency Medicine, Duke University Hospital, PO Box 3096, 2301 Erwin Road, Durham, NC 27110, USA; [b] Department of Emergency Medicine, Penn State Health Milton S. Hershey Medical Center, H043, 500 University Drive, Hershey, PA 17033, USA
* Corresponding author.
E-mail address: sreeja.natesan.md@gmail.com

Emerg Med Clin N Am 39 (2021) 733–744
https://doi.org/10.1016/j.emc.2021.08.001
emed.theclinics.com

There is also medicolegal risk associated with an incorrect or missed diagnosis and, more importantly, serious pathology that could lead to significant patient harm if not discovered.[2] A detailed history and physical examination is an excellent initial step, followed by the use of various laboratory and/or imaging studies to narrow the differential diagnosis.[1,5]

Common laboratory values frequently obtained in patients presenting to the ED with abdominal pain include complete blood count (CBC), electrolytes, amylase, lipase, liver enzymes, and urinalysis, but these may be of limited diagnostic value.[6] Some advocate against the overreliance on testing, including laboratory studies, as both normal and abnormal laboratory values may cause one to incorrectly diagnose or exclude certain diagnoses.[7] Despite extensive testing, the diagnosis may remain unclear and necessitate outpatient follow-up after initial ED evaluation through a primary care provider or referral to a specialist.[6] As early as 1994, an American College of Emergency Physicians policy statement recommended laboratory testing for only a few select diagnoses presenting with abdominal pain.[5] Others advise caution in certain populations, specifically the elderly, who often have a higher prevalence of significant pathology despite a reassuring examination and may warrant a broader workup than younger, healthier patients or those with fewer comorbidities.[7]

This caution regarding overutilization of laboratory testing must be balanced with ED throughput which impacts all patients presenting for care. Ordering a very limited medical evaluation and diagnostic testing from the waiting room was able to decrease several key throughput metrics in adult patients of similar triage levels presenting to the ED with abdominal pain.[8] If the cost of potential overordering is outweighed by the benefit of improved throughput, then one would want to focus on laboratory studies that maximize diagnostic value. The focus of this review will be to evaluate myriad laboratory studies that may be used to evaluate patients presenting with abdominal pain and other GI symptoms. It is important to note that tests range broadly in terms of sensitivity and specificity and may represent the causative problem or be a sequela of the pathology present and its associated symptoms.

GENERAL LABORATORY/PREOPERATIVE
Type and Screen/Type and Crossmatch

A type and screen is indicated in the setting of possible emergent transfusion or in preparation for potential surgical intervention. GI bleeding is a presentation to the ED that can range from mild and self-limiting to life-threatening. In patients with massive GI bleeding, uncrossmatched red blood cells may be transfused emergently.[9] Subsequent units of blood should be obtained after a blood type and screen has been sent and the patient has been appropriately crossmatched. This is also important in children presenting with GI bleeding, as the degree of blood loss associated with a Meckel's diverticulum can be quite profound.[10] However, routine ordering of a preoperative type and screen has been shown to be of low utility in common surgeries for abdominal pathology, such as appendectomy, cholecystectomy, and hernia repairs. A minimal increase in transfusion rates was seen among older patients compared to younger patients. Underlying medical conditions such as preexisting anemia, thrombocytopenia, or medical treatments such as anticoagulation may better predict the need for a transfusion than the specific type of procedure being performed.[11] It is important to take into consideration the anticipated findings, complications, and length of the procedure when determining if a preoperative type and screen with or without crossmatch is indicated. If a type and screen is not performed preoperatively and a transfusion is required, there always remains the option to provide uncrossmatched blood emergently or crossmatched blood obtained urgently.[11]

Complete Blood Count ± Differential

The CBC, with or without cell line differential, is one of the most commonly ordered tests, with focus primarily on the white blood cell count (WBC). However, the WBC may actually be one of the most contested laboratory tests of variable utility.[6] An elevated WBC in the context of abdominal pain may indicate serious pathology, although it is well noted to be neither sensitive nor specific in both adult and pediatric populations.[2,6,7] An example is how the reliance on the WBC is now limited in the setting of advanced imaging modalities for appendicitis in children.[10]

Demonstrating its unreliability, there is a portion of the population that has an elevated WBC at baseline, with a similar number of people having a baseline left shift of their WBC despite not having an active infection or abnormal pathology.[6] Conversely, patients can have a definitive diagnosis of pathology despite the absence of leukocytosis.[2,6,7] If possible, noting the trend of laboratory test results based on previous values may serve to determine if there is a true deviation from an individual's established baseline.

An abnormal WBC, while admittedly nonspecific, may be an indication of systemic illness with some clinical relevance for those presenting with abdominal pain.[5] In a retrospective analysis of patients presenting to an ED with abdominal pain, the presence of an elevated WBC demonstrated an association with having surgical pathology on univariate analysis, but this association was not found on multivariate analysis. No significant medical or surgical pathology was found in patients who lacked leukocytosis, lacked reports of vomiting on history, or possessed a reassuring abdominal examination without guarding or tachycardia on examination.[12] This further emphasizes the role of laboratory studies as adjuncts to a thorough history and physical examination.

An elevated WBC may raise the index of suspicion for certain conditions. If there is clinical concern of bowel obstruction, higher WBC values or the presence of a pronounced left shift was predictive of a serious pathology.[13] In the elderly, where the history and examination may be less reliable and the anticipated vital sign abnormalities may be blunted by comorbidities or concomitant medications, a CBC may be useful.[7] Owing to the change in T-cell function in the elderly, they are more prone to infection that is not evident by the mounting of fever or leukocytosis.[14]

Other elements of the CBC, namely the hemoglobin and hematocrit (H&H) and the platelet count, are equally important in the setting of GI bleeding. For patients that presented with complaints of dyspepsia, a normal H&H can be reassuring that there is no coexisting GI bleed.[15] Thrombocytopenia can also contribute to the severity of GI bleeding, and assessment of the platelet count, as a part of a coagulopathy workup, is also indicated.[9] GI bleeding that presents with anemia on arrival is associated with increased mortality particularly when the hemoglobin is less than 10 g/dL.[9] However, one should not be falsely reassured by a patient who is not initially anemic, as it may take up to a day for the extent of blood loss to become apparent via the H&H, especially with an acute episode of bleeding.[9] Serial H&H can be helpful to assess the true extent of blood loss and monitor ongoing bleeding.

Electrolytes, Blood Urea Nitrogen, and Creatine

While the name (basic metabolic panel [BMP], chemistry panel, renal panel, and so forth) and included elements may vary by manufacturer, the most common elements include electrolytes (ie, sodium, chloride, potassium, bicarbonate) and measures of kidney function, namely the blood urea nitrogen and creatinine. It is one of the more commonly ordered tests in the workup of abdominal pain, yet it is very nonspecific.[5] Although it is rarely diagnostic, this test may better reflect the sequelae of GI problems. Electrolytes and renal function should be assessed in patients with abdominal pain or cramping with associated vomiting and/or diarrhea. Suspicion of infectious diarrhea including bacterial, viral, or parasitic infections should prompt electrolyte and renal function testing. The water volume and electrolyte depletion can be quite profound with certain types of parasitic infection, such as *Cryptosporidium*, *Cystoisospora*, and *Giardia* species, especially in immunocompromised individuals.[16]

In pediatric patients with abrupt illnesses including malrotation or midgut volvulus, this test serves little diagnostic utility; however, it may show significant electrolyte derangement and evidence of failure to thrive in the setting of repeated vomiting in chronic intermittent malrotation without volvulus, which can be seen in older children and even adults.[10] Although corrected surgically, pyloric stenosis often requires significant medical resuscitation because of the profound electrolyte abnormalities and volume depletion associated with the repeated vomiting characteristic of this condition. Cases that have progressed beyond the earliest of stages may demonstrate the classic hypokalemic, hypochloremic metabolic alkalosis.[10] Therefore, children with recurrent, episodic, or progressive GI symptoms may benefit from a laboratory assessment of electrolytes and renal function.

INFLAMMATORY
Lactic Acid

Elevated lactate has been used to identify and assess a variety of conditions including sepsis, severity of trauma, malignancy, mesenteric ischemia, and pediatric cardiac disease, among others.[5,17] An elevated lactic acid may be useful for risk stratification, as those with varying degrees of elevated lactic acid levels have higher rates of morbidity and mortality, as has been demonstrated in critically ill patients with sepsis, other types of infection, as well as upper GI bleeding.[17] Regardless of the mechanism resulting in elevated lactate levels, one should consider it evidence of a metabolic injury. It can be a marker of hypoperfusion and end-organ damage before other more obvious clinical signs, such as hypotension.[17] While nonspecific, patients with an elevated lactic acid level should be prioritized to have focused interventions earlier in their clinical course to prevent further deterioration.[5] For example, in the setting of a small bowel obstruction, an elevated lactate level may be a marker of bowel ischemia.[13] Measuring a lactate is also warranted in the setting of GI bleeding. One recommendation is to use a threshold of 4 mmol/L to assist in risk stratification of the patient with GI bleeding early in their ED clinical course, as investigators demonstrated a 6.4-fold increased odds of mortality with measured lactate levels above this threshold value.[17] This same study also demonstrated a 1.4-fold increase in odds of mortality for every point increase in serum lactate levels, even when age, hematocrit upon presentation, and heart rate were controlled.[17]

C-Reactive Protein

The C-reactive protein (CRP) itself may not be independently diagnostic but is more discriminatory when the results coincide with other markers of inflammation or infection, such that the CRP and other laboratory values, such as WBC, are elevated or within normal limits.[18] This has been a suggested approach for several years. A 2004 meta-analysis supported the interpretation of CRP in conjunction with other historical, physical, and laboratory findings, rather than using a CRP in isolation.[18]

More recently, a prospective analysis of pediatric patients with acute appendicitis found that an elevated CRP (>3 mg/dL) found in conjunction with an elevated WBC (>12 cells × 1000/mm^3) demonstrated greater specificity than any independent measure.[19] These values can be particularly useful in younger pediatric patients who may not have a classic presentation similar to adults and have a higher misdiagnosis rate.[19]

Erythrocyte Sedimentation Rate

There is limited utility for erythrocyte sedimentation rate (ESR) in patients presenting to the ED with abdominal pain; however, it can be useful in some specific populations. In patients with an ulcerative colitis exacerbation, an elevated ESR in the setting of other clinical and laboratory abnormalities may indicate the need for admission.[20] ESR may have utility in the evaluation of pediatric patients with suspected functional pathology in which there remains diagnostic uncertainty; however, laboratory studies are considered low yield in the setting of a benign examination.[21] As early as the 1980s, the ESR was found to be of lesser value than the CRP and WBC in the diagnostic workup of children with histologically confirmed acute appendicitis. One study demonstrated that the ESR was only elevated in approximately 50% of patients symptomatic for ≥12 hours, and only 60% in patients with gangrenous and perforated appendicitis.[22]

Procalcitonin

Procalcitonin is a precursor to calcitonin secreted by the K cells of the lungs and the C cells of the thyroid.[1,23] Although typically undetectable in a normal individual, a cytokine-mediated inflammatory response can induce procalcitonin secretion in most parenchymal cells of the body.[23] The utility of procalcitonin in the setting of undifferentiated abdominal pain is still under investigation. It may serve a role in the management of small bowel obstructions, where it may indicate failure of conservative management and need for surgical intervention.[24] A systematic review found that this marker has high specificity for detecting complicated appendicitis but low sensitivity for uncomplicated appendicitis.[1,23]

INFECTIOUS
Blood Cultures

In cases of serious infection, blood cultures are often obtained to detect associated bacteremia. While it can be common practice to draw blood cultures in patients with certain clinical parameters, such as fever or leukocytosis, this often has limited utility. One study demonstrated that even in critically ill surgical patients, there was a low rate of positive blood cultures, approximately half of which were considered false positives. The authors concluded that routine blood cultures are of low yield, costly, rarely changed clinical management, and did not affect mortality and, therefore, advocated using them instead as a secondary measure of assessment.[25] Similar studies have demonstrated a low degree of utility for routine blood cultures in the ED.[26] However, it is prudent to recognize high-risk populations and specific diagnoses in which blood cultures may be beneficial. Patients at increased risk include the immunocompromised patients with cirrhosis, those with suspected bowel obstruction, and septic patients among others. Translocation of intestinal bacteria with associated sepsis has been noted in intestinal obstruction, particularly in immunocompromised and cirrhotic patients.[27–29] Blood cultures have been noted to be positive in 40% of cases of acute cholangitis.[30] Therefore, while blood cultures should not be considered a part of routine screening tests in abdominal pain, they should strongly be considered if the patient is noted to be at risk based on age or comorbidities, demonstrates signs of sepsis, or if certain infectious etiologies are suspected.

Stool Studies

Although not a routine part of ED evaluation for abdominal pain or diarrhea, stool studies may aid in the diagnosis in select scenarios. Identifying the nature of the likely infectious source, bacterial versus viral, is important in determining utility of stool studies or cultures.[31,32] The use of stool cultures should be reserved for severely ill or febrile patients or specific pediatric cases that warrant further investigation. The Wright stain, which detects fecal leukocytes, has a 52% to 82% sensitivity and 83% specificity for bacterial pathogen by stool culture, limiting its use in the routine workup of diarrhea.[33] Stool cultures are rarely helpful as they are only positive in 1% to 5% of cases.[32] Situations that may warrant stool culture include bloody or purulent diarrhea, community outbreaks, or in immunocompromised patient populations.[33,34] Clostridium difficile toxin assay may aid in evaluation of those patients with high-risk predisposition such as recent antibiotic use, recent hospitalization, immunocompromised status, or exposure.[33]

Parasitology Evaluation

With the increased ease and availability of travel and immersive experiences worldwide, obtaining a detailed history of potential exposures can help the clinician determine the risk of a parasitic infection. Parasitic infections should be considered in patients with travel histories, exposure to untreated water, or diarrhea persisting for more than 1 week.[33] Ova and parasite evaluation should be obtained in these patients, although multiple samples may need to be collected because of the intermittent shedding nature of parasites. Additional staining such as direct immunofluorescence may be used if Giardia or Cryptosporidium is suspected.[33] Parasitic infections can cause GI disease beyond diarrhea as well. While there are a multitude of parasitic diseases worldwide, we will focus this discussion on those found in the United States. **Table 1** lists the most common parasitic diseases with symptoms, incubation period, and special considerations.[35,36]

LIVER/BILIARY
Hepatic Function

Similar to the BMP discussed previously, a comprehensive metabolic panel includes the basic electrolytes and assessments of renal function but also assessments of the liver and biliary system. A hepatic function test includes liver markers such as aminotransferase levels (aspartate aminotransferase and alanine aminotransferase [ALT]), total bilirubin, total protein, albumin, and alkaline phosphatase and can help aid in diagnosis of primary versus secondary liver disease.[37] ALT is most specific for liver damage, although there is a poor correlation between the level and the extent of disease.[37] Serum gamma-glutamyl transferase (GGT) can be elevated in the setting of liver dysfunction, specifically obstructive biliary disease, as well as alcohol use.[38] Others advocate for its use as a biomarker for other disease processes, particularly chronic diseases such as heart and vascular disease, metabolic syndrome, cancer, and others.[38,39] While this list is not comprehensive, there is active research looking at its utilization in risk stratification for these chronic illnesses, given noticed trends by gender, ethnicity, and geography, which takes it beyond the scope of this review.[39]

Table 1
Parasitic causes of abdominal pain in the United States[35,36]

Disease Name	Parasite	Clinical Manifestation	Special Considerations
Chagas disease (American trypanosomiasis)	*Trypanosoma cruzi*	Acute infection within 4–8 wk of exposure • Romaña sign: swelling of the eyelid • Fever • Headache • Body aches • Rash • Loss of appetite • Vomiting/diarrhoea • Swelling at site of bite (chagoma) Chronic infection (up to 30% of patients) • Can result in heart conditions (arrhythmia, heart failure, risk of sudden death) and GI abnormalities (megaesophagus, megacolon)	• Mainly seen in rural Latin America, Mexico, & South America • Transmitted by triatomine bugs (kissing bug) that tend to bite people's faces and defecate on the wound • Also transmitted through congenital spread, blood transfusion, organ transplant • Blood donations are screened for the disease
Cyclosporiasis	*Cyclospora cayetanensis*	• Most common: Diarrhoea (watery) • Abdominal bloating and cramping • Increased flatulence • Fatigue, loss of appetite • Nausea • Weight loss	• Present on average 7 d (2 d to 2 wk) • Transmitted by consuming infected food or water • Most common in tropics/subtropical areas • Imported foods implicated: basil, cilantro, mesclun lettuce, raspberries, snow peas • Cyclospora oocytes are unlikely to be killed by routine sanitizing/chemical disinfection measures
Toxocariasis	*Toxocara*	• Typically asymptomatic until damage to affected organ Visceral infection: • Loss of appetite • Anemia • Fatigue • Fever • If lungs: coughing, wheezing	• Caused by roundworms from infected dog and cat feces or undercooked meat from infected animal • More common in hot/humid regions • Incubation period of 2–4 wk • Contamination occurs due to ingestion of

(continued on next page)

Table 1
(continued)

Disease Name	Parasite	Clinical Manifestation	Special Considerations
		• If abdomen: abdominal pain, hepatomegaly, anorexia • If brain: meningoencephalitis	*Toxocara* eggs (Eggs can survive for months-years out in the environment due to the strong outer layer.) • Eggs can travel through the bloodstream to different areas (brain, eyes, heart, lungs, liver, muscles).

The utility of GGT can also be questioned in the era of readily available advanced imaging and other laboratory testing. For example, it is sensitive in detecting the presence of liver disease, but it is not specific in determining the underlying etiology and can also be elevated in both acute and chronic conditions, such as pancreatitis, diabetes, alcohol abuse, and more.[38]

Coagulation studies including PT/PTT/INR and measures of specific coagulation factors can also be helpful in the assessment of liver disease. These laboratory values may be markers of overall liver synthetic function and suggest an underlying coagulopathy, which can be particularly helpful in the management of GI bleeding.[9]

Hepatitis Markers

In patients presenting to the ED with right upper quadrant pain, jaundice, or risk factors, testing for viral hepatitis can be helpful. Assessing the patient's symptoms and determining the nature and timing of the suspected exposure can help determine the likelihood of particular pathogens (**Table 2**).[40] Hepatitis B markers vary depending on the timing of infection. **Fig. 1** demonstrates the titers and time periods of expected positivity of various laboratory markers of Hepatitis B infection or vaccination over time.

Table 2
Viral hepatitis types and special considerations[40]

Type	Route of Transmission	Chronic Infection?	Prevention	Special Consideration
A	Fecal-oral	No	Immunization	
B	Blood/body fluids	Yes	Immunization	
C	Blood/body fluids	Yes	Blood donor screening program, decrease risk behavior	May lead to hepatocellular cancer or cirrhosis
D	Blood/body fluids	Yes	Immunization to hepatitis B; decrease in risk behavior	Needs coinfection with hepatitis B
E	Fecal-oral	No	Ensure sanitation & clean drinking water	High risk for pregnant patients

Marker	Acute Infection	Window Period	Chronic Infection	Cleared / Remote Infection	Immunization	Inactive Chronic Carrier
HBcAb	+	+	+	+	-	+
HBsAg	+	-	+	-	-	-
HBsAb	-	-	-	+	+	-

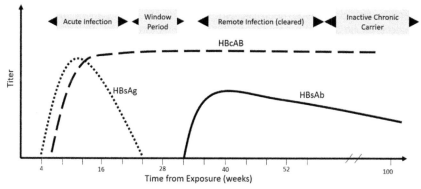

Fig. 1. Hepatitis B laboratory markers[40] titers and time periods of expected positivity of various laboratory markers of hepatitis B infection or vaccination over time. HBcAB, hepatitis B core antibody; HBsAb, hepatitis B surface antibody; HBsAg, hepatitis B surface antigen.

Ascitic Fluid Testing

Abdominal pain may be a manifestation of ascites with or without associated infection. The most common causes for ascites include underlying liver disease (viral hepatitis, sequelae of alcohol abuse, autoimmune disorders, and so forth), malignancy, and heart failure, followed by other less-frequent etiologies.[41] If a patient is presenting with new-onset ascites, a diagnostic paracentesis should be performed and fluid sent for cell count, culture, glucose, total protein, and albumin to help determine the etiology of the ascites. Tests for lactate dehydrogenase, amylase, and triglycerides and cytology may further help delineate the cause. A paracentesis should also be performed when considering spontaneous bacterial peritonitis (SBP), as SBP can be seen in approximately 15% of cirrhotic patients with ascites.[41]

PANCREATIC
Lipase and Amylase

Lipase and amylase are both commonly ordered in the workup of abdominal pain, with lipase being preferred as the diagnostic laboratory test of choice to evaluate for acute pancreatitis.[6,37] Despite its poor specificity, serum amylase was used frequently in the past in the assessment of pancreatitis as it was easy and cost-effective to measure. As the serum lipase value has proven itself more sensitive and specific to pancreatitis and become more affordable and widely available, it now supersedes serum amylase in the detection of acute pancreatitis.[15,42] While the specificity of lipase is superior to that of amylase, it is not perfect, and other conditions may contribute to an elevated lipase level, such as other GI issues (ie, appendicitis, cholecystitis, peritonitis, small bowel obstruction, and more) and tumors that produce lipolytic enzymes, hypertriglyceridemia, trauma, and others.[15,42,43] Diabetics have been shown to have a higher baseline serum lipase value, likely secondary to certain oral hypoglycemic agents, and so the threshold for interpretation may require adjustment.[15,44] In the setting of chronic pancreatitis, the clinical picture is further clouded, as both the serum amylase and lipase levels are decreased, with serum amylase decreased to a greater extent.[43] It is important to note that the degree of amylase and/or lipase elevation does not necessarily correlate with the severity of disease, nor should it be used for trending clinical response.

Contrast-enhanced CT is the preferred imaging modality to assess for severity of pancreatitis and pancreatic necrosis. Not required of every patient, the utility of advanced imaging should be guided by the clinical picture of the patient.[5] If the presentation is not clearly consistent with pancreatitis, the laboratory measures are not diagnostic, or there is concern for a complication of pancreatitis, one should consider pursuing imaging with contrast-enhanced CT.[5,15]

SUMMARY

As abdominal pain is one of the most common presenting complaints to the ED, a clear understanding of the nuances of the indications and reliability of available laboratory tests can help the ED care provider in the workup of this patient population. Laboratory testing should serve as an adjunct to the history and physical examination to narrow down the broad differential diagnosis of abdominal complaints. The combination of these can help guide patient care while allocating resources appropriately and being mindful of ED throughput, efficiency, and patient safety measures.

CLINICS CARE POINTS

- Abdominal pain and vomiting are two of the most common chief complaints seen in emergency departments across the country.
- Laboratory testing should be focused and guided by the history, physical examination, and working differential diagnosis.
- Caution should be used with populations who are at higher risk of pathology, such as the elderly and immunocompromised. These patients may require a broader diagnostic workup including laboratory evaluation and diagnostic imaging.

DISCLOSURE

No disclosures to report.

REFERENCES

1. Natesan S, Lee J, Volkamer H, et al. Evidence-based medicine approach to abdominal pain. Emerg Med Clin North Am 2016;34(2):165–90.
2. Macaluso CR, McNamara RM. Evaluation and management of acute abdominal pain in the emergency department. Int J Gen Med 2012;5:789–97.
3. Rui P, Kang K. National Hospital Ambulatory Medical care survey: 2017 emergency department summary tables. National Center for Health Statistics. Available at: https://www.cdc.gov/nchs/data/nhamcs/web_tables/2017_ed_web_tables-508.pdf. Accessed October 26, 2020.

4. Bhuiya FA, Pitts SR, McCaig LF. Emergency department visits for chest pain and abdominal pain: United States, 1999-2008. NCHS Data Brief 2010;(43):1–8.
5. Panebianco NL, Jahnes K, Mills AM. Imaging and laboratory testing in acute abdominal pain. Emerg Med Clin North Am 2011;29(2):175–93, vii.
6. Graff LG 4th, Robinson D. Abdominal pain and emergency department evaluation. Emerg Med Clin North Am 2001;19(1):123–36.
7. Kamin RA, Nowicki TA, Courtney DS, et al. Pearls and pitfalls in the emergency department evaluation of abdominal pain. Emerg Med Clin North Am 2003; 21(1):61–72, vi.
8. Begaz T, Elashoff D, Grogan TR, et al. Initiating diagnostic studies on patients with abdominal pain in the waiting room decreases time spent in an emergency department bed: a randomized controlled trial. Ann Emerg Med 2017;69(3): 298–307.
9. Nable JV, Graham AC. Gastrointestinal bleeding. Emerg Med Clin North Am 2016;34(2):309–25.
10. D'Agostino J. Common abdominal emergencies in children. Emerg Med Clin North Am 2002;20(1):139–53.
11. Ghirardo SF, Mohan I, Gomensoro A, et al. Routine preoperative typing and screening: a safeguard or a misuse of resources. JSLS 2010;14(3):395–8.
12. Abbas SM, Smithers T, Truter E. What clinical and laboratory parameters determine significant intra abdominal pathology for patients assessed in hospital with acute abdominal pain? World J Emerg Surg 2007;2:26.
13. Nagarwala J, Dev S, Markin A. The vomiting patient: small bowel obstruction, cyclic vomiting, and gastroparesis. Emerg Med Clin North Am 2016;34(2):271–91.
14. Leuthauser A, McVane B. Abdominal pain in the geriatric patient. Emerg Med Clin North Am 2016;34(2):363–75.
15. Robinson P, Perkins JC Jr. Approach to patients with epigastric pain. Emerg Med Clin North Am 2016;34(2):191–210.
16. Garcia LS, Arrowood M, Kokoskin E, et al. Practical guidance for clinical microbiology laboratories: laboratory diagnosis of parasites from the gastrointestinal tract. Clin Microbiol Rev 2017;31(1):e00025-17.
17. Shah A, Chisolm-Straker M, Alexander A, et al. Prognostic use of lactate to predict inpatient mortality in acute gastrointestinal hemorrhage. Am J Emerg Med 2014;32(7):752–5.
18. Andersson RE. Meta-analysis of the clinical and laboratory diagnosis of appendicitis. Br J Surg 2004;91(1):28–37.
19. Kwan KY, Nager AL. Diagnosing pediatric appendicitis: usefulness of laboratory markers. Am J Emerg Med 2010;28(9):1009–15.
20. Carlberg DJ, Lee SD, Dubin JS. Lower abdominal pain. Emerg Med Clin North Am 2016;34(2):229–49.
21. Smith J, Fox SM. Pediatric abdominal pain: an emergency medicine perspective. Emerg Med Clin North Am 2016;34(2):341–61.
22. Peltola H, Ahlqvist J, Rapola J, et al. C-reactive protein compared with white blood cell count and erythrocyte sedimentation rate in the diagnosis of acute appendicitis in children. Acta Chir Scand 1986;152:55–8.
23. Yu CW, Juan LI, Wu MH, et al. Systematic review and meta-analysis of the diagnostic accuracy of procalcitonin, C-reactive protein and white blood cell count for suspected acute appendicitis. Br J Surg 2013;100(3):322–9.
24. Cosse C, Regimbeau JM, Fuks D, et al. Serum procalcitonin for predicting the failure of conservative management and the need for bowel resection in patients with small bowel obstruction. J Am Coll Surg 2013;216(5):997–1004.

25. Henke PK, Polk HC Jr. Efficacy of blood cultures in the critically ill surgical patient. Surgery 1996;120(4):752–9.
26. Kelly AM. Clinical impact of blood cultures taken in the emergency department. Emerg Med J 1998;15:254–6.
27. Vaishnavi C. Translocation of gut flora and its role in sepsis. Indian J Med Microbiol 2013;31(4):334–42.
28. Riordan SM, Williams R. The intestinal flora and bacterial infection in cirrhosis. J Hepatol 2006;45(5):744–57.
29. Wiest R, Garcia-Tsao G. Bacterial translocation (BT) in cirrhosis. Hepatology 2005;41(3):422–33.
30. Sokal A, Sauvanet A, Fantin B, et al. Acute cholangitis: diagnosis and management. J Visc Surg 2019;156(6):515–25.
31. DuPont HL. Acute infectious diarrhea in immunocompetent adults. N Engl J Med 2014;370(16):1532–40.
32. Gale AR, Wilson M. Diarrhea: initial evaluation and treatment in the emergency department. Emerg Med Clin North Am 2016;34(2):293–308.
33. Kman NE, Werman HA. Disorders presenting primary with diarrhea. In: Tintinalli JE, Stapczynski JS, Cline DM, et al, editors. Tintinalli's emergency medicine: a comprehensive study guide. 7th edition. New York: McGraw-Hill; 2011. p. 531–40.
34. Graves NS. Acute gastroenteritis. Prim Care 2013;40(3):727–41.
35. CDC - Parasites - Neglected parasitic infections (NPIs) in the United States. Centers for disease control and prevention. Available at: https://www.cdc.gov/parasites/npi/index.html. Accessed February 1, 2021.
36. Woodhall D, Jones JL, Cantey PT, et al. Neglected parasitic infections: what every family physician needs to know. American Family Physician. Available at: https://www.aafp.org/afp/2014/0515/p803.html#afp20140515p803-t1.   Accessed February 1, 2021.
37. Avegno J, Carlisle M. Evaluating the patient with right upper quadrant abdominal pain. Emerg Med Clin North Am 2016;34(2):211–28.
38. Whitfield JB. Gamma glutamyl transferase. Crit Rev Clin Lab Sci 2001;38(4):263–355.
39. Koenig G, Seneff S. Gamma-glutamyltransferase: a predictive biomarker of cellular antioxidant inadequacy and disease risk. Dis Markers 2015;2015:818570.
40. Viral hepatitis tools for health professionals. Centers for Disease Control and Prevention. 2020. Available at: https://www.cdc.gov/hepatitis/resources/healthprofessionaltools.htm. Accessed February 6, 2021.
41. Hou W, Sanyal AJ. Ascites: diagnosis and management. Med Clin North Am 2009;93(4):801–vii.
42. Smith RC, Southwell-Keely J, Chesher D. Should serum pancreatic lipase replace serum amylase as a biomarker of acute pancreatitis? ANZ J Surg 2005;75(6):399–404.
43. Yadav D, Agarwal N, Pitchumoni CS. A critical evaluation of laboratory tests in acute pancreatitis. Am J Gastroenterol 2002;97(6):1309–18.
44. Jones MR, Hall OM, Kaye AM, et al. Drug-induced acute pancreatitis: a review. Ochsner J 2015;15(1):45–51.

Approach to Abdominal Imaging in 2022

Daniel S. Brenner, MD, PhD[a],*, Tiffany C. Fong, MD[b]

KEYWORDS

- Ultrasound • POCUS • CT • MRI • Abdominal pain

KEY POINTS

- Ultrasonography can be used as a focused screening tool for abdominal pathology.
- Iodinated contrast is safe in patients with GFR greater than 30.
- In the evaluation of patients with abdominal pain, CT is often the first-line imaging study, but MRI is an alternative for select patients.

INTRODUCTION

Abdominal pain represents 5% to 7% of all emergency department (ED) presentations.[1,2] Many patients require imaging for diagnosis, and choosing the appropriate imaging modality is a crucial decision point. Modern medicine offers a broad array of options including abdominal x-ray (AXR), computed tomography (CT), MRI, and ultrasonography. This article introduces the commonly available modalities, discusses the advantages and disadvantages, and presents current recommendations.

Abdominal x-ray

AXR is an inexpensive, commonly available modality. Although AXR involves significantly less radiation exposure than CT, it lacks sufficient sensitivity or specificity for routine use.[3,4] AXR has been used in pediatric populations to screen for high-risk diagnoses and evaluate for constipation despite evidence suggesting that this approach lacks sensitivity and can delay critical diagnoses.[5] AXR does have utility to identify radiopaque ingested foreign bodies and in the emergent evaluation for small bowel obstruction or perforation before a confirmatory study.[6]

Abdominal computed tomography

Abdominal CT is one of the most versatile and impactful imaging tools.[7,8] This tool provides excellent data on bony structures and solid organs but can miss subtle intestinal

---

[a] Department of Emergency Medicine, 3rd Floor FOB, 720 Eskenazi Ave, Indianapolis, IN 46202, USA; [b] Department of Emergency Medicine, Johns Hopkins School of Medicine, 1830 East Monument Street, Suite 6-100, Baltimore, MD 21287, USA
* Corresponding author.
E-mail address: dsbrenne@iu.edu

Emerg Med Clin N Am 39 (2021) 745–767
https://doi.org/10.1016/j.emc.2021.07.007

pathology such as fistulae. The examination is brief enough that people with claustrophobia can usually tolerate it. Drawbacks including radiation exposure (estimated 3–10 mSv per CT abdomen/pelvis) and cost (estimated $1000–3000 per scan) prevent CT from being used universally.[4,9] The true lifetime-associated risk of cancer from CT radiation exposure is controversial. Linear scaling of data from major exposures (Hiroshima, Chernobyl) to CT-associated dose exposures suggest that scanning 1000 individuals may cause one additional case of cancer, but there are few epidemiologic studies to validate this prediction.[10] One such recently published study did demonstrate a slightly increased incidence of hematological malignancy in patients who underwent CT abdomen/pelvis to evaluate for appendicitis.[11]

Intravenous (IV) injection of iodinated contrast improves the diagnostic accuracy of CT and enhances the appearance of inflammation. Contrast can be timed to highlight arterial structures (CT angiography [CTA]) or venous structures.[12] Oral or rectal contrast can be administered to better evaluate intestinal pathology, but improvements in CT resolution have made this unnecessary except in the evaluation of abnormal intestinal architecture including gastric bypass/resections, fistulae, or anastomotic leaks.[13]

Classically, use of IV iodinated contrast has been limited by concerns for contrast-induced nephropathy (CIN), defined as a worsening of renal function after administration of iodinated contrast. However, the existence and severity of CIN is controversial, and data suggest that CIN is rare with the use of modern contrast agents.[14,15] Recent consensus statements recommend that IV contrast may be used without limitation in patients with glomerular filtration rate (GFR) greater than 45 and may be used with consideration of prophylactic volume expansion with isotonic fluids in patients with GFR 30 to 45.[16,17] Although data suggest that iodinated contrast may even be safe for use in patients with GFR 15 to 30 and in some patients with minimal renal function who are not dialysis dependent, this is still controversial. Discussion with specialists is recommended before contrast administration in these patients unless contrast is necessary for a time-sensitive critical diagnosis.

Iodine "allergies" can be another barrier to administration of iodinated contrast, but pure iodine is a chemical element that is essential to life and cannot be an allergen.[18] These reactions should be recategorized as either anaphylactoid non-IgE-mediated reactions to iodinated contrast media that require pretreatment or nonspecific reactions that do not require pretreatment (shellfish allergies, skin reactions to topical iodine-based antiseptics).[18] Anaphylactoid reactions to iodinated contrast are feared but rare (0.6% of exposures), and severe reactions are extremely uncommon (0.04% of exposures).[19] Evidence-based pretreatment regimens are 12- to 24-hour protocols,[20] which are ill-suited for use in the ED. Truncated protocols (methylprednisolone 40 mg or hydrocortisone sodium succinate 200 mg 4 hours before the scan, diphenhydramine 50 mg 1 hour before scan) have been developed but not validated.[12,21]

Abdominal Ultrasonography

Ultrasonography is a versatile tool in the diagnosis of abdominal pathology. This technique offers rapid, low-cost bedside evaluation without radiation exposure. Ultrasonography can be performed by ultrasonographers and interpreted by radiologists or can be performed at the bedside and interpreted by trained emergency physicians (point-of-care ultrasound [POCUS]). Ultrasonography tends to be a highly specific diagnostic tool that sometimes lacks sensitivity. Ultrasound waves cannot pass through air, limiting evaluation of bowel or structures deep to bowel. Image quality is also hindered by greater depths of tissue, which attenuate sound waves. When used properly, it can expedite diagnosis and reduce cost and radiation exposure but cannot always independently exclude diagnoses.

The accuracy of ultrasonography depends highly on the user's skill, because inexperienced users may be unable to obtain adequate images. Despite this limitation, evidence suggests that ultrasonographic competence can be rapidly acquired with supervised practice.[22]

Abdominal MRI

MRI can also be used for the evaluation of abdominal complaints, although it is rarely used in the ED. MRI provides excellent soft tissue contrast resolution for a wide range of diagnoses and may be especially useful in pediatric or pregnant patients to avoid radiation exposure.[23] MRI can be enhanced with the administration of gadolinium-based contrast, but this should be avoided in patients with GFR less than 30 to avoid potentially devastating nephrogenic systemic fibrosis. Notably, there is no allergic cross-reactivity between iodine-based and gadolinium-based contrasts.

The use of emergency abdominal MRI is limited by several factors. MRI examinations incur considerable expense relative to diagnostic films, ultrasonography, or even CT. Although ultrafast MRI protocols have been developed, many abdominal protocols require 45 to 90 minutes and complete immobility. Patients may struggle with claustrophobia and require anxiolysis or sedation. Emergency MRI use is also limited by availability; even tertiary facilities may not have around-the-clock availability.

RECOMMENDATIONS FOR ABDOMINAL IMAGING BY ABDOMINAL REGION

The remainder of this article summarizes the available evidence for imaging in abdominal diagnoses, organized by region. Although regional localization of pain in the abdomen is imperfect, it provides a useful schema in considering critical diagnoses.[24] Keeping a broad differential in patients with abdominal pain and applying imaging modalities according to clinical pretest probability will lead to efficient and effective care.

Right Upper Quadrant Pain

Biliary

Biliary disease (including cholecystitis, cholangitis, and choledocholithiasis) is common.[25] Historical and physical examination findings of biliary pathology are unreliable, with factors such as fever (sensitivity 44%–62%, specificity 37%–50%), emesis (sensitivity 83%, specificity 56%), right upper quadrant pain (sensitivity 47%–93%, specificity 0%–96%), and Murphy sign (sensitivity 62%, specificity 96%) insufficient for reliable diagnosis.[26]

The American College of Radiology recommends ultrasonography for biliary pathology (**Table 1**).[27,28] Findings suggestive of cholecystitis include cholelithiasis, anterior gallbladder wall thickness greater than 3 mm, pericholecystic fluid, and dilated common bile duct greater than 4 mm (or 10% of the patient's age) (**Fig. 1**).[29] The sonographic Murphy sign (pain with inspiration with the probe on the gallbladder) has excellent specificity (95%) but poor sensitivity (66%).[29] Of note, critically ill patients often have incidental abnormal ultrasonographic findings that do not correlate with true biliary pathology.[30]

If ultrasonographic findings are equivocal, the clinician should consider following with CT with IV contrast, ^{99m}Tc-labeled hepatobiliary iminodiaceteic acid (HIDA) scintigraphy, or MRI.[27] Although CT is commonly available its sensitivity may be relatively low and it is unreliable in the diagnosis of cholesterol-based cholelithiasis.[28,31] HIDA

Table 1
Test characteristics for right upper quadrant pathology

	Ultrasonography (Sens/Spec)		CT (Sens/Spec)		MRI/MRCP (Sens/Spec)		HIDA (Sens/Spec)	
Cholecystitis	82%	81%	94%	59%	86%	82%	94%	90%
Biliary obstruction	55%–95%	71%–96%	74%–96%	90%–94%	93%	NR	NR	NR

Abbreviations: HIDA, ^{99m}Tc-labeled hepatobiliary iminodiaceteic acid; MRCP, magnetic resonance cholangiopancreatography; NR, not reported; Sens, sensitivity; Spec, specificity.

scan assesses uptake of an IV radioactive tracer by hepatocytes and the rate of tracer excretion into the gallbladder as bile. Cystic duct blockage causes decreased tracer entry into the gallbladder and is diagnostic of cholecystitis.[28] Although HIDA has excellent diagnostic power, it is a technically challenging study that can take hours to perform and is potentially confounded by prestudy administration of opioids.[32] MRI is also sensitive and specific for cholecystitis and is better able to identify gallstones and biliary tract inflammation than CT.[28,33] With administration of contrast, MRI may also be able to differentiate between acute and chronic cholecystitis.[34]

Painless jaundice
Painless jaundice is uncommon and is usually associated with intrahepatic cholestasis or mechanical obstruction (choledocholithiasis, neoplasm, or biliary stricture). If clinical suspicion favors choledocholithiasis, ultrasonography is recommended for initial evaluation because it is effective at identifying biliary ductal dilation. However, if the presentation is more concerning for stricture or neoplasm, CT with contrast and MRI with magnetic resonance (MR) cholangiopancreatography (MRCP) are reasonable alternatives.[35] CT can often identify neoplastic causes of biliary stricture, but may miss small pancreatic head masses or intraductal neoplasms.[35] MRCP provides optimal visualization of the biliary tree and has excellent sensitivity for biliary obstruction and malignancy.[36] In the ED, initial screening with CT is often sufficient as long as outpatient follow-up can be arranged.

Portal vein thrombosis
Portal vein thrombosis is thrombosis or embolism of the trunk of the portal vein. This condition generally presents with nonspecific symptoms including transient abdominal pain, fever, nausea, and diarrhea but can also be completely asymptomatic; it is relatively rare in the general population but can be associated with cirrhosis, pancreatitis, prothrombotic disorders, or malignancy. Ultrasonography, CT with contrast, and MRI are all appropriate for diagnosis (**Fig. 2**), and POCUS diagnosis of portal vein thrombosis has also been reported.[37]

Epigastric Pain

Dyspepsia
Most causes of dyspepsia are benign, but upper gastrointestinal (GI) malignancy is an important but uncommon cause.[38] Features including age greater than 60 years, family history of upper GI malignancy, weight loss, dysphagia, persistent vomiting, palpable mass, or jaundice have traditionally been indications for upper endoscopy. Younger patients from regions with high prevalence of gastric cancer (Southeast Asia, South America) may also merit endoscopy.[39] Patients with classic symptoms of dyspepsia do not require imaging in the ED.

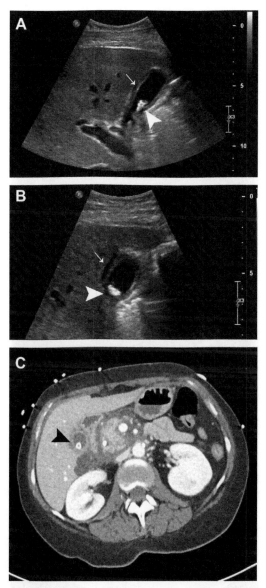

Fig. 1. Cholecystitis. Longitudinal (*A*) and transverse (*B*) ultrasound windows demonstrating cholelithiasis (*arrowhead*) with pericholecystic fluid (*arrows*) and gallbladder wall thickening (*arrows*). Axial CT image (*C*) demonstrating cholelithiasis (*arrowhead*) with pericholecystic fluid.

Acute pancreatitis

Acute pancreatitis is the leading cause of hospitalization among GI disorders and most commonly results from gallstones and alcohol use.[40,41] Disease severity may range from mild pancreatitis to infected necrosis with multiorgan dysfunction.[42]

Most cases can be diagnosed based on typical symptoms and laboratory studies alone, without the need for imaging. Impaired pancreatic perfusion and necrosis

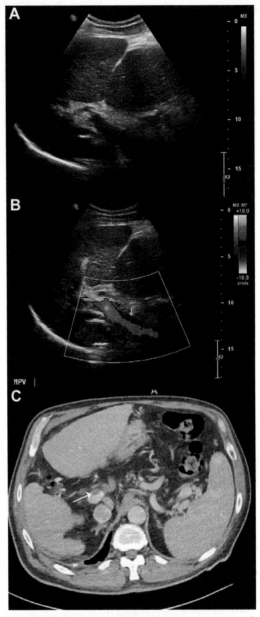

Fig. 2. Portal vein thrombosis. Ultrasonography demonstrating portal vein (*A*) with color Doppler (*B*) demonstrating lack of flow suggesting thrombus (*green arrow*). CT demonstrating portal vein thrombosis (*C, white arrow*).

evolve over days, and early imaging correlates poorly with disease severity, seldom changes management, and does not improve clinical outcomes.[43,44] In typical acute pancreatitis, biliary ultrasonography should be used to screen for culprit gallstones. Unfortunately, sonographic assessment of the pancreas is limited. Abnormal findings are seen in as low as 33% of ultrasonographic studies, including pancreatic enlargement, hypoechoic edematous tissue, or peripancreatic fluid.[45]

For patients with *atypical* pancreatitis with equivocal lipase, American College of Radiology recommends CT abdomen with IV contrast.[46] Typical CT findings include diffuse or localized edematous enlargement of the pancreas, stranding of the peripancreatic fat, peripancreatic free fluid, and discrete fluid collections (**Fig. 3**). Although noncontrast CT abdomen can also identify these findings, IV contrast enhances the ability to identify pancreatic necrosis and stratify disease severity.[28]

Abdominal MRI, like CT, has a limited role to diagnose or assess the severity of pancreatitis in the acute setting. However, MRCP is both sensitive and specific for choledocholithiasis and may help identify those who require urgent endoscopic retrograde cholangiopancreatography.[47] The soft tissue contrast resolution of MRI offers superior pancreatic imaging but does not adequately evaluate bowel if there is concern for intestinal pathology.

Local complications of pancreatitis

Pancreatic or peripancreatic necrosis is distinguishable from nonnecrotic fluid collections after 5 to 7 days of symptoms.[42] Acute peripancreatic fluid collections usually do not require intervention, because half of the fluid collections resolve spontaneously over weeks.[48] CT abdomen with IV contrast is the most common initial test to evaluate fluid collections but is not ideal to identify and quantify debris or to differentiate pseudocysts (managed through endoscopic techniques; see **Fig. 3**) from walled-off necrosis (requiring possible surgical debridement). MRI is the best modality to assess for necrosis of peripancreatic collections.

Left Upper Quadrant Pain

Splenic disorders

Splenic pathology (including infection, atraumatic rupture, malignancy, aneurysm) is a relatively rare cause of left upper quadrant pain. CT abdomen with IV contrast is effective in characterizing splenic lesions. Unenhanced CT can miss certain lesions that are isodense with the spleen. Although ultrasonography can identify some focal splenic lesions, findings are often nonspecific and frequently require CT for further characterization. MRI evaluates the spleen well, but not significantly better than CT.

Right Lower Quadrant Pain

Appendicitis

Appendicitis is estimated to represent 4% of the presentations for acute abdominal pain.[49] The classic symptoms and signs including migratory pain, Rovsing sign, and obturator sign are specific but not sensitive.[50] For this reason, suspicion of acute appendicitis usually requires radiologic evaluation.

Ultrasonography can be used to screen for acute appendicitis (**Table 2**).[51] An ultrasonographic study demonstrating definitive acute appendicitis (outer diameter >6 mm, noncompressible, periappendiceal free fluid, luminal fecolith) (**Fig. 4**) does not require confirmatory imaging.[52] A negative or inconclusive ultrasonographic evaluation is common in adults, particularly in pregnant patients.[53] Intriguingly, retrospective data in pediatric patients suggest that patients with an inconclusive ultrasonography and a white blood cell count less than 7.5×10^9/L have a negative predictive value of 97%.[54]

A nondiagnostic ultrasonography should prompt additional imaging, typically CT with IV contrast.[41] Findings suggestive of appendicitis on CT include a dilated tubular structure stemming from the cecum with associated inflammation (see **Fig. 3**).

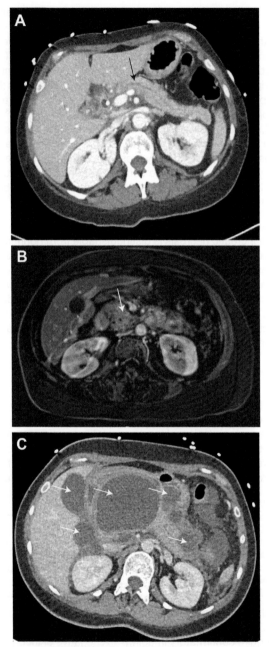

Fig. 3. Pancreatitis. CT (*A*) and MRI (*B*) demonstrating pancreatic inflammation and edema (*arrows*). CT (*C*) demonstrating multiple large pancreatic pseudocysts (*white arrows*).

Although oral contrast was previously recommended for the evaluation of appendicitis, this is no longer necessary.[55] A small body of evidence suggests that noncontrast CT may be useful in the diagnosis of acute appendicitis in patients who are unable to tolerate contrast.[56]

Table 2
Test characteristics for right lower quadrant pathology

	Ultrasonography (Sens/Spec)	Radiography (Sens/Spec)	CT (Sens/Spec)	MRI (Sens/Spec)
Appendicitis	84% 91%	0% NR	91% 90%	97% 95%
Epiploic appendagitis	NR NR	NR NR	NR NR	NR NR

Abbreviations: NR, Not reported; Sens, sensitivity; Spec, specificity.

MRI has not been well studied in the diagnosis of appendicitis, but preliminary studies suggest that MRI has high sensitivity and specificity with similar findings.[57] If available, MRI is an appealing option in the evaluation of pregnant and pediatric populations to avoid exposure to ionizing radiation.

Epiploic appendagitis
Epiploic appendagitis is caused by torsion of an epiploic appendage on the colon leading to appendage thrombosis and necrosis. This condition typically presents with sudden severe abdominal pain and can mimic conditions such as appendicitis, cholecystitis, and diverticulitis but does not generally require intervention.[58] Ultrasonography, CT, and MRI all seem to be sufficient for diagnosis with findings that include an oval hyperechoic, noncompressible mass with surrounding inflammatory changes.[58]

Left Lower Quadrant Pain

Diverticulitis
In Western countries, diverticulitis usually presents with left lower quadrant (LLQ) pain due to preferential involvement of the descending and sigmoid colon.[59] Although

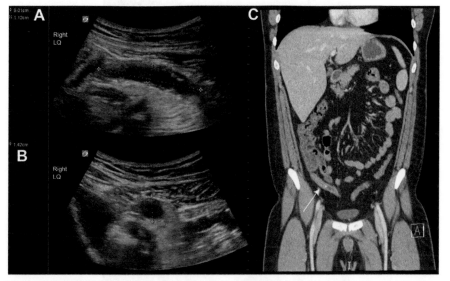

Fig. 4. Appendicitis. Longitudinal (*A*) and transverse (*B*) ultrasound views demonstrating a dilated appendix with periappendiceal fluid. CT (*C*) demonstrating appendicitis (*white arrow*) with appendicolith and periappendiceal inflammation.

diverticulitis can be diagnosed without imaging in patients with typical signs and symptoms, imaging is frequently pursued to confirm the diagnosis, assess the extent of disease, and identify complications (**Fig. 5**).

The American College of Radiology recommends CT abdomen and pelvis with IV contrast for patients with LLQ pain.[60] The use of IV contrast permits detection of subtle bowel wall abnormalities, as well as diverticular abscesses. Oral contrast does not add diagnostic benefit.[61] Water-soluble (to avoid barium peritonitis) rectal contrast may be administered to evaluate for leak or perforation following a surgical intervention.

Alternative modalities to assess for diverticulitis include MRI and ultrasonography (**Table 3**). MRI performs well to diagnose acute diverticulitis and can identify associated abscess or colonic neoplasm.[60] However, the ability to identify extraluminal air from a perforation is more limited. Abdominal ultrasonography with graded compression may be diagnostic for uncomplicated diverticulitis but performs poorly in complicated diverticulitis.[62] Fluoroscopy with contrast enema is no longer recommended but may be helpful in follow-up to evaluate for fistulas, strictures, and to assist in surgical planning.

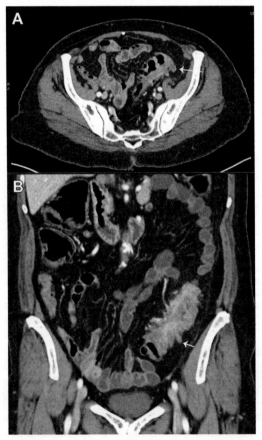

Fig. 5. Diverticulitis. Axial (*A*) and coronal (*B*) CT demonstrating diverticuli (*arrows*) with thickened, inflamed bowel wall.

Flank Pain

Nephrolithiasis

Patients typically present with acute-onset flank pain and hematuria but often require imaging for initial diagnosis. Ultrasonography can be used as a primary screening tool in patients with high likelihood of nephrolithiasis (**Table 4**). POCUS findings of hydronephrosis (**Fig. 6**) and absence of ureteric jets in the bladder has good sensitivity with moderate specificity, and POCUS reduces radiation exposure without worsening outcomes.[63] For patients with an equivocal ultrasonography and high pretest probability for nephrolithiasis, CT abdomen/pelvis without contrast is appropriate to visualize high-density calculi. If there is concern for alternative pathology, CT abdomen/pelvis with contrast is also acceptable. Findings on CT include ureteral stone with evidence of hydronephrosis and/or ureteral inflammation (see **Fig. 6**). In patients who cannot undergo CT, MRI is a reasonable alternative with good sensitivity and excellent specificity.[64] Although some groups recommend AXR for follow-up of previously diagnosed renal stones, it is a not an appropriate ED test for nephrolithiasis.[65]

Pyelonephritis

Uncomplicated patients with pyelonephritis do not require imaging.[66] For complicated patients with concern for perinephric abscess or emphysematous pyelonephritis, CT with contrast is recommended.[67] Although 3-phase contrast was previously recommended, single-phase nephrographic scans are now sufficient (**Fig. 7**).[67] MRI is a viable alternative for patients who cannot undergo CT imaging, with excellent sensitivity and specificity even without contrast, although contrast enhancement is preferred.[53] Ultrasonography should not be used to assess for pyelonephritis, because the sensitivity is unacceptably low.[68]

Pelvic/Groin Pain

Female pelvic pain

The first-line modality for pain of a suspected gynecologic or obstetric cause in premenopausal women is transabdominal or transvaginal ultrasonography.[69] A transabdominal technique provides a larger field of view but less detail than transvaginal ultrasonography. CT can diagnose renal/urologic causes of pelvic pain as well as gynecologic pathology. MRI may also identify these findings but is discouraged as an initial test given the time-sensitive nature of these diagnoses.

Ovarian torsion

Transvaginal ultrasonography is the preferred diagnostic modality for ovarian torsion (**Table 5**). Sonographic evidence of ovarian torsion includes ovarian enlargement and edema with variable Doppler findings including absent, decreased, or reversed ovarian arterial flow. Abnormal venous flow seems to have the highest sensitivity and specificity for torsion.[70] A "whirlpool sign" may be seen, representing a twisted ovarian vascular pedicle. CT with contrast can also evaluate for ovarian torsion, with findings including an enlarged ovary with lack of enhancement, ovarian

Table 3							
Test characteristics for left lower quadrant pathology							
	Ultrasound (Sens/Spec)		Radiography (Sens/Spec)		CT (Sens/ Spec)		MRI (Sens/ Spec)
Diverticulitis	77%–98%	80%–99%	0%		NR	97%	93% 86%–94% 88%–92%

Abbreviations: NR, not reported; Sens, sensitivity; Spec, specificity.

Table 4
Test characteristics for flank pathology

	Ultrasonography (Sens/Spec)		Radiography (Sens/Spec)		CT (Sens/Spec)		MRI (Sens/Spec)	
Nephrolithiasis	84%	53%	58%	69%	97%	96%	82%	98%
Pyelonephritis	33%	85%	0%	NR	90%	96%	95%	95%

Abbreviations: NR, not reported; Sens, sensitivity; Spec, specificity.

hematoma, twisted vascular pedicle, thickened fallopian tube, surrounding fat stranding, and free fluid. Although data in this topic are limited, ovarian torsion seems to be unlikely in the setting of normal ovarian size on CT.[71] Given the limited diagnostic performance of radiological studies, in select patients with high pretest probability for ovarian torsion there should be consideration of diagnostic laparoscopy even with reassuring ultrasonography or CT.

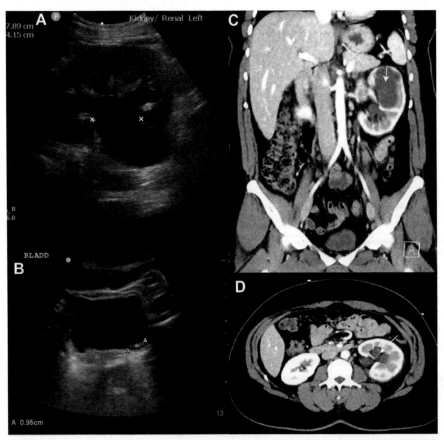

Fig. 6. Nephrolithiasis. Moderate hydronephrosis (*A*) with dilation of the renal pelvis and proximal calices. Nephrolith (*B*) at the ureterovesciular junction. Coronal (*C*) and axial (*D*) CT views of left sided moderate hydronephrosis (*white arrows*). UVJ, uretovesicular junction.

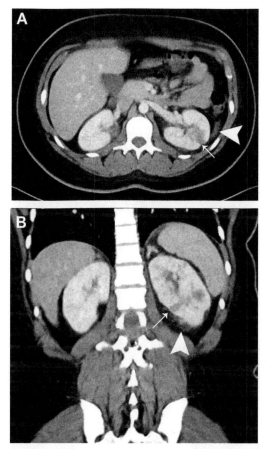

Fig. 7. Pyelonephritis. Axial (*A*) and coronal (*B*) CT views of pyelonephritis with wedge-shaped infarct (*arrow*) and perinephric inflammation (*arrowheads*).

Ectopic pregnancy

Ultrasonography is the recommended initial study in the evaluation for ectopic pregnancy, with excellent sensitivity and specificity.[72] In cases in which ultrasonography

Table 5
Test characteristics for pelvic pathology

	Ultrasonography (Sens/Spec)		CT (Sens/Spec)		MRI (Sens/ Spec)	
Ovarian torsion	70%	87%	100%	NR	85%	83%
Ruptured ovarian cyst	NR	99%	NR	NR	NR	NR
Tubo-ovarian abscess	56%–93%	86%–98%	78%–100%	75%–82%	NR	NR
Testicular torsion	94%	98%	NR	NR	NR	NR
Torsion of testicular appendage	57%	100%	NR	NR	NR	NR
Ectopic pregnancy	98%	99%	NR	NR	NR	NR

Abbreviations: NR, not reported; Sens, sensitivity; Spec, specificity.

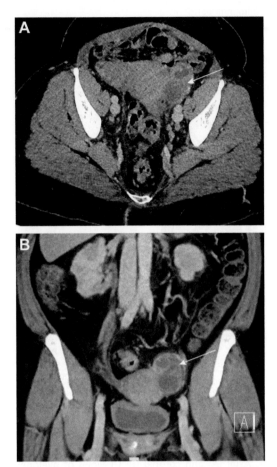

Fig. 8. Hydrosalpinx. Axial (*A*) and coronal (*B*) CT views of the dilated fluid-filled fallopian tube (*white arrows*).

is nondiagnostic or unavailable, expert opinion suggests that both CT and MRI are appropriate for the diagnosis of ectopic or heterotopic pregnancy, although MRI is preferred given the risk of irradiating pregnant women.[73] In unstable patients, laparoscopy is the preferred diagnostic and therapeutic modality.

Upper genital tract infection

Pelvic inflammatory disease (PID) is a clinical diagnosis that does not require imaging and often has no sonographic abnormalities. In atypical or severe presentations, PID can be visualized as thickened or hypervascular fallopian tube (**Fig. 8**). With progression to salpingitis or tubo-ovarian abscess (**Fig. 9**), a hyperemic, solid, or cystic adnexal mass becomes visible. CT with oral and IV contrast has higher sensitivity than ultrasonography to detect tubo-ovarian abscess, but acutely ill patients often cannot tolerate the oral contrast or wait for the contrast to progress to the distal bowel.[74,75]

Male pelvic pain

An acute scrotum, characterized by testicular pain and scrotal swelling, requires emergent imaging. The most concerning cause is testicular torsion, requiring

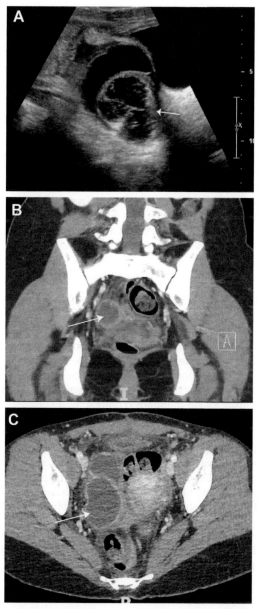

Fig. 9. Tubo-ovarian abscess. Transvaginal ultrasonography (*A*) demonstrating cystic loculated mass (*white arrow*) contiguous with the left ovary. Coronal (*B*) and axial (*C*) CT images demonstrating cystic lobulated structure (*white arrows*) associated with left ovary.

diagnosis and intervention within 6 hours to prevent ischemia and necrosis. Ultrasonography of the scrotum with Doppler is the best imaging modality for all acute scrotal complaints, with high diagnostic accuracy.[76] In testicular torsion, ultrasonography can identify twisting of the spermatic cord with high-resistance arterial waveforms.

Table 6
Test characteristics for nonlocalized pathology

	Ultrasonography (Sens/Spec)		Radiography (Sens/Spec)		CT (Sens/Spec)		MRI (Sens/Spec)	
Bowel obstruction	87%	75%	49%	98%	93%	93%	95%	100%
Ingested foreign body	NR	NR	90%	100%	NR	NR	NR	NR
Peritoneal abscess	75%	91%	NR	NR	88%	93%	NR	NR

Abbreviations: NR, not reported; Sens, sensitivity; Spec, specificity.

The most common cause of acute scrotal symptoms is epididymitis. Epididymitis manifests as an enlarged epididymis with hypervascularity on Doppler, often associated with scrotal wall edema and reactive hydrocele. In prepubertal boys, torsion of the testicular appendage is the most common cause of scrotal pain but is difficult to see on ultrasonography and requires only supportive management.

CT and MRI are rarely used to evaluate acute scrotal abnormalities, although they are potentially helpful when ultrasonography is inconclusive.

Nonlocalized Pain

Severe nonlocalized pain (peritonitis) is thought to represent activation of the visceral peritoneal afferent fibers. The differential for diffuse pain is extremely broad and often necessitates imaging.

CT abdomen/pelvis with contrast is the recommended first study, because it offers rapid and broad evaluation (**Table 6**).[77] If the pretest probability for vascular pathology is high, CTA is preferred. Noncontrast CT can also be used in patients who cannot receive iodinated contrast, but if the noncontrast imaging is nondiagnostic and there is high pretest probability for life-threatening pathology, a contrasted CT study or MRI can be considered.[77] Modern MRI scanners can reduce the acquisition time, and one prospective study demonstrated excellent performance in the diagnosis of a wide range of abdominal pathology.[59]

Although AXR is rapidly available, the sensitivity for most diagnoses is extremely low and AXR should not delay the acquisition of definitive imaging.[77]

Ultrasonography is capable of diagnosing many pathologic entities but is not recommended for unfocused examinations. Ultrasonography is best used to test for a specific diagnosis, because complete ultrasonographic abdominal examinations are time consuming and inefficient.[77] In limited resource situations without access to cross-sectional imaging, ultrasonography can be considered in the evaluation of diffuse abdominal pain.

Table 7
Test characteristics for vascular pathology

	Ultrasonography (Sens/Spec)		Radiography (Sens/Spec)		CT (Sens/Spec)		MRI (Sens/Spec)	
Aortic dissection/ aneurysm	94%	98%	NR	NR	100%	100%	96%	100%
Mesenteric ischemia	NR	NR	NR	NR	93%	96%	NR	NR

Abbreviations: NR, not reported; Sens, sensitivity; Spec, specificity.

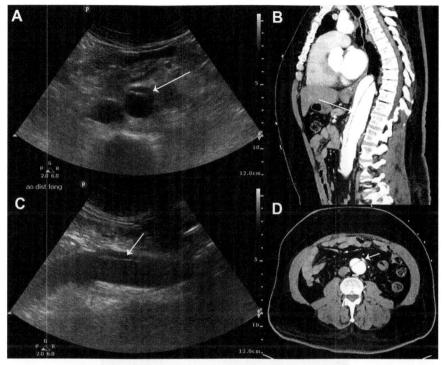

Fig. 10. Aortic dissection. Transverse (*A*) and longitudinal (*C*) ultrasonographic views of the aorta demonstrating a dissection flap (*white arrows*). Sagittal (*B*) and axial (*D*) CTA views demonstrating dissection flap (*white arrows*).

Vascular Catastrophe

Aortic aneurysm/dissection

Aortic pathology is difficult to diagnose because both dissection and aneurysm frequently present with atypical symptoms and require high clinical suspicion guiding appropriate imaging.

CTA is the recommended diagnostic imaging study for aortic dissection and aneurysm (**Table 7**).[78] Findings of dissection include intimal flap, double lumen, aortic dilatation, intramural hematoma, and findings of aneurysm include dilatation greater than 3 cm (**Figs. 10** and **11**). Noncontrast CT may be able to identify pathologic conditions with findings including high-density mural hematoma and displacement of atherosclerotic calcification into the lumen[79] but has an unacceptably low false-negative rate. Rapid-protocoled MRI also has excellent sensitivity and specificity, but is still slower, more expensive, and less available than CTA.[80]

Ultrasonography, including POCUS, is also highly sensitive and specific for abdominal aortic aneurysm and dissection.[81] Common protocols include an examination of the proximal, middle, and distal aorta assessing for dissection flap, aortic dilatation greater than 3 cm, and intraluminal clot (see **Fig. 11**). In unstable patients with concern for aortic pathology, it is reasonable to perform an immediate abdominal POCUS examination followed by emergent CTA.

Mesenteric ischemia

Mesenteric ischemia classically presents with abdominal pain out of proportion with examination and nonspecific abdominal symptoms. CTA is the recommended study

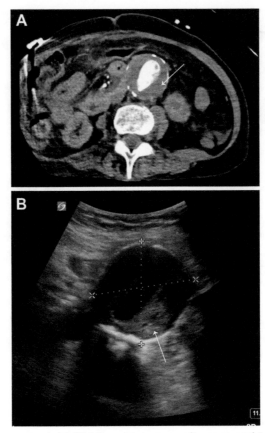

Fig. 11. Aortic aneurysm. Axial CT (*A*) and transverse ultrasonographic (*B*) views demonstrating aortic aneurysm with associated thrombus (*white arrows*).

to evaluate mesenteric ischemia[82] with findings including arterial stenosis, bowel wall thickening/dilation, mesenteric fat stranding, pneumatosis intestinalis, and portal vein gas. Data on the use of MRI in acute mesenteric ischemia are sparse and conflicted.[83] In patients who have an absolute contraindication to CTA, MRI/MR angiography may be considered.

Ultrasonography can identify areas of bowel ischemia suggestive of mesenteric ischemia, and duplex studies can identify clots in the proximal mesenteric vessels. However, these studies cannot reliably exclude the diagnosis. Therefore, ultrasonography may be used as a screening tool to expedite diagnosis but should not delay a definitive study.

DISCLOSURE

The authors have nothing to disclose.

REFERENCES

1. Powers RD, Guertler AT. Abdominal pain in the ED: stability and change over 20 years. Am J Emerg Med 1995;13(3):301–3.

2. Hastings RS, Powers RD. Abdominal pain in the ED: A 35 year retrospective. Am J Emerg Med 2011;29(7):711–6.
3. Smith JE, Hall EJ. The use of plain abdominal x rays in the emergency department. Emerg Med J 2009;26(3):160–3.
4. Hart D, Wall BF. UK population dose from medical X-ray examinations. Eur J Radiol 2004;50(3):285–91.
5. Ferguson CC, Gray MP, Diaz M, et al. Reducing unnecessary imaging for patients with constipation in the pediatric emergency department. Pediatrics 2017;140(1): e20162290.
6. Tseng HJ, Hanna TN, Shuaib W, et al. Imaging foreign bodies: ingested, aspirated, and inserted presented at the American roentgen ray society annual meeting, Toronto, Ontario, Canada, April 2015. Ann Emerg Med 2015;66(6): 570–82.e5.
7. Acr–Spr Practice Parameter for the Performance of Computed Tomography (Ct) of the Abdomen and Computed Tomography (Ct) of the Pelvis. Am Coll Radiol 2014;1076:1–18.
8. Pandharipande PV, Reisner AT, Binder WD, et al. CT in the emergency department: a real-time study of changes in physician decision making. Radiology 2016;278(3):812–21.
9. Brenner DJ, Hall EJ, Phil D. Computed tomography-an increasing source of radiation exposure. vol. 357. 2007. Available at: www.nejm.org.
10. National Academy of Sciences: Washington, DC. National research council (NRC) to assess health risks from exposure to low levels of ionizing radiation: BEIR VIII phase 2. 2006.
11. Lee KH, Lee S, Park JH, et al. Risk of hematologic malignant neoplasms from abdominopelvic computed tomographic radiation in patients who underwent appendectomy. JAMA Surg 2021;156(4):343–51.
12. ACR Committee on drugs and contrast Media. ACR manual on contrast media. vol. 105.; 2013. Available at: http://www.acr.org/~/media/ACR/Documents/PDF/QualitySafety/Resources/Contrast Manual/2013_Contrast_Media.pdf.
13. Jensen CT, Blair KJ, Le O, et al. Utility of CT oral contrast administration in the emergency department of a quaternary oncology hospital: diagnostic implications, turnaround times, and assessment of ED physician ordering. Abdom Radiol 2017;42(11):2760–8.
14. Hinson JS, Ehmann MR, Fine DM, et al. Risk of acute kidney injury after intravenous contrast media administration. Ann Emerg Med 2017;69(5):577–86.e4.
15. Bucher AM, de Cecco CN, Schoepf UJ, et al. Is contrast medium osmolality a causal factor for contrast-induced nephropathy? Biomed Res Int 2014;2014: 931413.
16. Hinson JS, Ehmann MR, Klein EY. Evidence and patient safety prevail over myth and dogma : consensus guidelines on the use of intravenous contrast media. Ann Emerg Med 2020;76(2):149–52.
17. Davenport MS, Perazella MA, Yee J, et al. Use of intravenous iodinated contrast media in patients with kidney disease: consensus statements from the American College of Radiology and the National Kidney Foundation. Radiology 2020; 294(2):660–8.
18. Schabelman E, Witting M. The relationship of radiocontrast, iodine, and seafood allergies: a medical myth exposed. J Emerg Med 2010;39(5):701–7.
19. Wang CL, Cohan RH, Ellis JH, et al. Frequency, outcome, and appropriateness of treatment of nonionic iodinated contrast media reactions. AJR Am J Roentgenol 2008;191(2):409–15.

20. Lasser EC, Berry CC, Mishkin MM, et al. Pretreatment with corticosteroids to prevent adverse reactions to nonionic contrast media. AJR Am J Roentgenol 1994; 162(3):523–9.

21. Mervak BM, Cohan RH, Ellis JH, et al. Intravenous corticosteroid premedication administered 5 hours before CT compared with a traditional 13-hour oral regimen. Radiology 2017;285(2):425–33.

22. Gibson LE, White-Dzuro GA, Lindsay PJ, et al. Ensuring competency in focused cardiac ultrasound: a systematic review of training programs. J Intensive Care 2020;8(1):93.

23. Yu HS, Gupta A, Soto JA, et al. Emergency abdominal MRI: current uses and trends. Br J Radiol 2016;89(1061):1–12.

24. Morley EJ, Bracey A, Reiter M, et al. Association of pain location with computed tomography abnormalities in emergency department patients with abdominal pain. J Emerg Med 2020;59(4):485–90.

25. Shaffer EA. Epidemiology of gallbladder stone disease. Best Pract Res Clin Gastroenterol 2006;20(6):981–96.

26. Jain A, Mehta N, Secko M, et al. History, physical examination, laboratory testing, and emergency department ultrasonography for the diagnosis of acute cholecystitis. Acad Emerg Med 2017;24(3):281–97.

27. Peterson CM, McNamara MM, Kamel IR, et al. ACR appropriateness criteria ® right upper quadrant pain. J Am Coll Radiol 2019;16(5):S235–43.

28. Kiewiet JJS, Leeuwenburgh MMN, Bipat S, et al. A systematic review and meta-analysis of diagnostic performance of imaging in acute cholecystitis. Radiology 2012;264(3):4–129.

29. Hilsden R, Leeper R, Koichopolos J, et al. Point-of-care biliary ultrasound in the emergency department (BUSED): implications for surgical referral and emergency department wait times. Trauma Surg Acute Care Open 2018;3(1):1–5.

30. Boland GW, Slater G, Lu DS, et al. Prevalence and significance of gallbladder abnormalities seen on sonography in intensive care unit patients. AJR Am J Roentgenology 2000;174(4):973–7.

31. Patel NB, Oto A, Thomas S. Multidetector CT of emergent biliary pathologic conditions. Radiographics 2013;33(7):1867–88.

32. Cervellin G, Mora R, Ticinesi A, et al. Epidemiology and outcomes of acute abdominal pain in a large urban Emergency Department: retrospective analysis of 5,340 cases. Ann Translational Med 2016;4(19):362.

33. Tonolini M, Ravelli A, Villa C, et al. Urgent MRI with MR cholangiopancreatography (MRCP) of acute cholecystitis and related complications: diagnostic role and spectrum of imaging findings. Emerg Radiol 2012;19(4):341–8.

34. Wang A, Shanbhogue AK, Dunst D, et al. Utility of diffusion-weighted MRI for differentiating acute from chronic cholecystitis. J Magn Reson Imaging 2016; 44(1):89–97.

35. Lalani T, Couto CA, Rosen MP, et al. ACR appropriateness criteria jaundice. J Am Coll Radiol 2013;10(6):402–9.

36. Hakansson K, Ekberg O, Hakansson HO, et al. MR and ultrasound in screening of patients with suspected biliary tract disease. Acta Radiol 2002;43:80–6.

37. Wells D, Brackney A. Acute portal vein thrombosis diagnosed with point-of-care ultrasonography. Clin Pract Cases Emerg Med 2017;1(1):50–2.

38. Eusebi LH, Black CJ, Howden CW, et al. Effectiveness of management strategies for uninvestigated dyspepsia: systematic review and network meta-analysis. BMJ 2019;367:l6483.

39. Moayyedi PM, Lacy BE, Andrews CN, et al. ACG and CAG clinical guideline: management of dyspepsia. Am J Gastroenterol 2017;112(7):988–1013.
40. Yadav D, Lowenfels AB. The epidemiology of pancreatitis and pancreatic cancer. Gastroenterology 2013;144(6):1252–61.
41. Peery AF, Dellon ES, Lund J, et al. Burden of gastrointestinal disease in the United States: 2012 update. Gastroenterology 2012;143(5):1179–87.e3.
42. Banks PA, Bollen TL, Dervenis C, et al. Classification of acute pancreatitis - 2012: Revision of the Atlanta classification and definitions by international consensus. Gut 2013;62(1):102–11.
43. Kothari S, Kalinowski M, Kobeszko M, et al. Computed tomography scan imaging in diagnosing acute uncomplicated pancreatitis: usefulness vs cost. World J Gastroenterol 2019;25(9):1080–7.
44. Reynolds PT, Brady EK, Chawla S. The utility of early cross-sectional imaging to evaluate suspected acute mild pancreatitis. Ann Gastroenterol 2018;31(5): 628–32.
45. Balthazar EJ. Acute pancreatitis: assessment of severity with clinical and CT evaluation. Radiology 2002;223(3):603–13.
46. Porter KK. ACR appropriateness Criteria® acute pancreatitis. J Am Coll Radiol 2019. https://doi.org/10.1016/j.jacr.2019.05.017.
47. Meeralam Y, Al-Shammari K, Yaghoobi M. Diagnostic accuracy of EUS compared with MRCP in detecting choledocholithiasis: a meta-analysis of diagnostic test accuracy in head-to-head studies. Gastrointest Endosc 2017;86(6):986–93.
48. Patra PS, Das K. Vascular complications of acute pancreatitis. Clin Gastroenterol Hepatol 2014;12(12):2136–7.
49. Benabbas R, Hanna M, Shah J, et al. Diagnostic accuracy of history, physical examination, laboratory tests, and point-of-care ultrasound for pediatric acute appendicitis in the emergency department: a systematic review and meta-analysis. Acad Emerg Med 2017;24(5):523–51.
50. Lee SH, Yun SJ. Diagnostic performance of emergency physician-performed point-of-care ultrasonography for acute appendicitis: a meta-analysis. Am J Emerg Med 2019;37(4):696–705.
51. Lembcke B. Ultraschalldiagnostik der akuten appendizitis - so sieht's aus: 30 Jahre fundierte Ultraschalldiagnostik der Appendizitis - eine visuelle Philippika zu Praxis, Pittoreskem, Problemen und Potenzial. Z Gastroenterol 2016;54(10): 1151–65.
52. Smith MP, Katz DS, Lalani T, et al. ACR appropriateness criteria \ right lower quadrant PainVSuspected appendicitis 2015. Available at: http://journals.lww.com/ultrasound-quarterly.
53. Williams R, Shaw J. Ultrasound scanning in the diagnosis of acute appendicitis in pregnancy. Emerg Med J 2007;24(5):359.
54. Cohen B, Bowling J, Midulla P, et al. The non-diagnostic ultrasound in appendicitis: is a non-visualized appendix the same as a negative study? J Pediatr Surg 2015;50:923–7.
55. Farrell CR, Bezinque AD, Tucker JM, et al. Acute appendicitis in childhood: oral contrast does not improve CT diagnosis. Emerg Radiol 2018;25(3):257–63.
56. Lane MJ, Liu DM, Huynh MD, et al. Suspected acute appendicitis: nonenhanced helical CT in 300 consecutive patients 1. Radiology 1999;213:341–6.
57. Barger RL, Nandalur KR. Diagnostic performance of magnetic resonance imaging in the detection of appendicitis in adults. A meta-analysis. Acad Radiol 2010; 17(10):1211–6.

58. Giannis D, Matenoglou E, Sidiropoulou MS, et al. Epiploic appendagitis: pathogenesis, clinical findings and imaging clues of a misdiagnosed mimicker. Ann Transl Med 2019;7(24):814.
59. Imaeda H, Hibi T. The burden of diverticular disease and its complications: west versus east. Inflamm Intestinal Dis 2018;3(2):61–8.
60. Galgano SJ, Mcnamara MM, Peterson CM, et al. ACR appropriateness criteria ® 2 left lower quadrant pain-suspected diverticulitis left lower quadrant pain-suspected diverticulitis expert Panel on gastrointestinal imaging. J Am Coll Radiol 2019 May; 16(5s): S141-S149.
61. Kessner R, Barnes S, Halpern P, et al. CT for acute nontraumatic abdominal pain—is oral contrast really required? Acad Radiol 2017;24(7):840–5.
62. Nielsen K, Richir MC, Stolk TT, et al. The limited role of ultrasound in the diagnostic process of colonic diverticulitis. World J Surg 2014;38(7):1814–8.
63. Smith-Bindman R, Aubin C, Bailitz J, et al. Ultrasonography versus Computed Tomography for Suspected Nephrolithiasis. N Engl J Med 2014;371(12):1100–10.
64. Brisbane W, Bailey MR, Sorensen MD. An overview of kidney stone imaging techniques. Nat Rev Urol 2016;13(11):654–62.
65. Mutgi A, Williams JW, Nettleman M. Renal colic utility of the plain abdominal roentgenogram. Available at: https://jamanetwork.com/.
66. Nikolaidis P, Dogra VS, Goldfarb S, et al. ACR appropriateness criteria® acute pyelonephritis. J Am Coll Radiol 2018;15(11):S232–9.
67. Taniguchi LS, Torres US, Souza SM, et al. Are the unenhanced and excretory CT phases necessary for the evaluation of acute pyelonephritis? Acta Radiol 2017; 58(5):634–40.
68. Yoo JM, Koh JS, Han CH, et al. Diagnosing acute pyelonephritis with CT, 99mTc-DMSA SPECT, and Doppler ultrasound: a comparative study. Korean J Urol 2010; 51(4):260–5.
69. Bhosale PR, Javitt MC, Atri M, et al. ACR appropriateness Criteria® acute pelvic pain in the reproductive age group 2016. Available at: http://journals.lww.com/ultrasound-quarterly.
70. Grunau GL, Harris A, Buckley J, et al. Diagnosis of ovarian torsion: is it time to forget about doppler? J Obstet Gynaecol Can 2018;40(7):871–5.
71. Moore C, Meyers AB, Capotasto J, et al. Prevalence of abnormal CT findings in patients with proven ovarian torsion and a proposed triage schema. Emerg Radiol 2009;16(2):115–20.
72. Ong CL, Wong L, Yang Y, et al. Accuracy of ultrasonography in detecting ectopic pregnancy. Ultrasound Med Biol 2017;43:S140.
73. Kao LY, Scheinfeld MH, Chernyak V, et al. Beyond ultrasound: CT and MRI of ectopic pregnancy. AJR Am J Roentgenology 2014;202(4):904–11.
74. Hiller N, Fux T, Finkelstein A, et al. CT differentiation between tubo-ovarian and appendiceal origin of right lower quadrant abscess: CT, clinical, and laboratory correlation. Emerg Radiol 2016;23(2):133–9.
75. Lee DC, Swaminathan AK. Sensitivity of ultrasound for the diagnosis of Tubo-Ovarian abscess: a case report and literature review. J Emerg Med 2011;40(2): 170–5.
76. Ota K, Fukui K, Oba K, et al. The role of ultrasound imaging in adult patients with testicular torsion: a systematic review and meta-analysis. J Med Ultrason 2019; 46(3):325–34.
77. Scheirey CD, Fowler KJ, Therrien JA, et al. ACR Appropriateness Criteria ® acute nonlocalized abdominal pain. J Am Coll Radiol 2018;15(11):S217–31.

78. Sebastià C, Pallisa E, Quiroga S, et al. Aortic dissection: diagnosis and follow up with helical CT. Radiographics 1999;19:45–60.
79. Kurabayashi M, Okishige K, Ueshima D, et al. Diagnostic utility of unenhanced computed tomography for acute aortic syndrome. Circ J 2014;78(8):1928–34.
80. Panting JR, Norell MS, Baker C, et al. Feasibility, accuracy and safety of magnetic resonance imaging in acute aortic dissection safety of magnetic resonance imaging in acute aortic dissection. Clin Radiol 1995;50(7):455–8.
81. Costantino TG, Bruno EC, Handly N, et al. Accuracy of emergency medicine ultrasound in the evaluation of abdominal aortic aneurysm. J Emerg Med 2005;29(4):455–60.
82. Jan M. Diagnostic accuracy of multidetector CT in acute mesenteric ischemia: systematic review and meta-analysis. Radiology 2010;256(1):93–101.
83. Ginsburg M, Obara P, Lambert DL, et al. ACR appropriateness criteria® imaging of mesenteric ischemia. J Am Coll Radiol 2018;15(11):S332–40.

Avoiding Misdiagnosis of Abdominal Vascular Catastrophes

David C. Snow, MD, MSc[a],*, Kristi Colbenson, MD[b]

KEYWORDS

- Blunt abdominal trauma • Penetrating abdominal trauma • Bowel ischemia
- Abdominal aortic aneurysm • Aortic occlusion

KEY POINTS

- The increased availability of advanced imaging modalities has helped decrease mortality of traumatic abdominal vascular injuries over time, but the clinician should have an organized and diligent approach to these patients to prevent both missed injury and unexpected decompensation.
- Despite accounting for the minority of vascular injuries, blunt trauma is responsible for 80% of deaths due to unreliable signs and symptoms as well as difficulty diagnosing concomitant injuries to other organ systems.
- Bowel ischemia can occur acutely due to occlusion of intestinal arteries or veins, or it can be nonocclusive in low perfusion states. Clinical suspicion in the elderly followed by emergent computed tomography angiography helps minimize diagnosis delays.
- Acute embolic mesenteric ischemia is optimally managed by a multidisciplinary team to allow for hybrid endovascular and open procedure to restore flow.
- The management of abdominal aortic aneurysm rupture includes timely diagnosis, permissive hypotension, and transfer to a facility that can perform endovascular or open repair.
- Abdominal aortic aneurysm endograft complications include endograft leak, angulation kinking, migration, and thrombosis.

ABDOMINAL VASCULAR ANATOMY

The abdomen is a cylinder-like chamber extending from the inferior portion of the thorax to the superior portion of the pelvis. It can be divided into the peritoneal cavity, retroperitoneal cavity, and pelvis. The retroperitoneum is surrounded anteriorly by the parietal peritoneum and posteriorly by the transversalis fascia. The major blood

[a] Loyola University Medical Center, 2160 S. First Avenue, Maywood, IL 60153, USA; [b] Mayo Clinic, 2204 Baihly Vista Ln SW, Rochester, MN 55902, USA
* Corresponding author.
E-mail address: David.c.snow@lumc.edu

Emerg Med Clin N Am 39 (2021) 769–780
https://doi.org/10.1016/j.emc.2021.08.002   emed.theclinics.com
0733-8627/21/© 2021 Elsevier Inc. All rights reserved.

vessels of the abdomen are contained within this space, including the abdominal aorta, inferior vena cava, superior mesenteric artery (SMA), inferior mesenteric artery (IMA), and renal arteries.

The aorta gives rise to several paired and unpaired vessels within the abdomen. The paired arteries (adrenal, renal, and gonadal) provide blood supply to their respective organs. The unpaired arteries (celiac, SMA, and IMA) deliver blood to the gastrointestinal tract, spleen, gallbladder, pancreas, and liver. The celiac trunk branches off of the aorta at 90° and is thus less susceptible to embolic phenomena than the SMA and IMA.

The 3 branches of the celiac trunk (splenic, left gastric, and common hepatic arteries) supply the foregut structures from the distal esophagus to the second part of the duodenum, the spleen, the liver, and parts of the pancreas (**Fig. 1**). The SMA arises just below the celiac trunk and gives rise to several branches that supply blood to the midgut, from the second portion of the duodenum to the distal third of the transverse colon. The SMA branches from the aorta at approximately the level of the first lumbar vertebrae. The IMA arises just proximal to the aortic bifurcation, at approximately the level of the fourth lumbar vertebrae, and supplies blood to the hindgut, extending from the transverse colon to the rectum (**Fig. 2**).

The venous system of the gastrointestinal tract differs from the arterial system in that, rather than draining into the inferior vena cava (IVC), it passes via the portal vein into the liver. Blood passes through the hepatic lobules into the hepatic veins, which then pass into the IVC.[1]

TRAUMATIC ABDOMINAL VASCULAR EMERGENCIES

Abdominal vascular trauma presents many challenges to the treating clinician. These injuries can be lethal and are more commonly associated with penetrating rather than blunt trauma. The most commonly injured vessels are the aorta, SMA, iliac arteries, IVC, portal vein, and iliac veins.[2]

Abdominal vascular injuries rarely occur in isolation. It is thought that 2 to 4 associated intraabdominal injuries occur with each vascular injury.[2] It is for this reason that many of the signs and symptoms associated with solid organ injury are considered when evaluating for vascular injury.

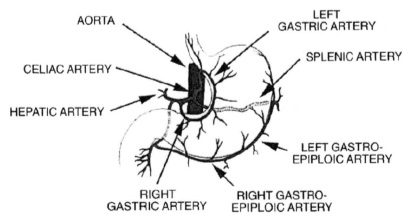

Fig. 1. The celic artery and its 3 majors branches: the splenic, left gastric, and hepatic arteries. (*Data from* Walkers JS, Dire DJ. Vascular abdominal emergencies. Emerg Med Clin North Am 1996;14(3):573; with permission.)

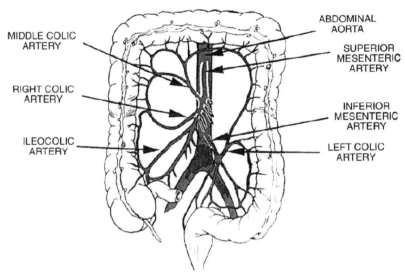

Fig. 2. The superior and inferior mesenteric arteries and their anastomotic connections. (*Data from* Walkers JS, Dire DJ. Vascular abdominal emergencies. Emerg Med Clin North Am 1996;14(3):573; with permission.)

Mortality from abdominal vascular injuries remains high, with 20% to 60% noted from a combination of exsanguination and multisystem organ failure.[3] The increased availability of advanced imaging modalities has helped decrease mortality over time, but the clinician should have an organized and diligent approach to these patients to prevent both missed injury and unexpected decompensation.

Mechanism—Blunt Trauma

Blunt trauma accounts for most of the trauma patients seen in emergency departments. Most of these injuries are caused by motor vehicle collisions, whereas some are caused by falls and direct blows. Despite accounting for the minority of vascular injuries (5%–40%), blunt trauma is responsible for most of the deaths (80%)[4,5] due to unreliable signs and symptoms as well as difficulty diagnosing concomitant injuries to other organ systems.

Traumatic injuries can occur through several possible mechanisms: seatbelts can compress the abdomen when exposed to abrupt deceleration; sudden increases in intraabdominal pressure can rupture hollow organs; direct trauma can compress the abdomen against the vertebrae or thoracic cage injuring solid organs (most commonly the spleen and liver); and shearing forces from the deceleration can lacerate both hollow and solid organs alike. Vascular structures within the abdomen are at risk with any of these injuries.

Mechanism—Penetrating Trauma

Within the spectrum of penetrating trauma, stabbing and ballistic mechanisms are the most common. Stab wounds cause damage by laceration and tearing, whereas the higher energy of gunshot wounds also causes damage to the surrounding tissue it penetrates by temporary cavitation. Despite stabbings being 3 times more common, firearms cause almost 90% of the deaths, mainly due to the greater energy that is transmitted to tissues.[6] As with blunt trauma, organs are more likely injured than vascular structures, with small intestine, colon, and liver injuries occurring most frequently. However, penetrating trauma does account for 60% to 95% of vascular abdominal injuries.[4] Importantly, as much as 30% of penetrating chest trauma may traverse the diaphragm and also injure intraabdominal structures, so a heightened suspicion is needed with penetrating injuries to the lower thoracic cavity.[7]

Initial Evaluation

The initial presentation for those with a vascular traumatic injury ranges from hemodynamic stability to profound shock. The hemodynamic stability of the patient largely depends on whether the injury has resulted in tamponade (eg, a contained retroperitoneal hematoma) or is freely rupturing into the peritoneal cavity.

For vascular injury, the clinical features are nonspecific, including abdominal pain, abdominal distention, back or flank pain, or the expected findings of hemorrhagic shock including hypotension and tachycardia. Bruising to the flank (Grey-Turner sign) may indicate retroperitoneal bleeding, but this finding is both a nonspecific and potentially delayed finding (~12 hours).

The presence of a seat-belt sign, rebound tenderness, abdominal distention, or guarding all raise the likelihood of an intraabdominal injury, although these are not specific to vascular injuries. It is worthwhile to note that the lack of abdominal tenderness on examination does not rule out an intraabdominal injury.[8]

Hemorrhage within the pelvis can be catastrophic if not found early, with unexplained hypotension being the only indication. Instability of the pelvic ring should be considered in those with blunt trauma with possible pelvic fractures, and a pelvic binder is a priority in the management of the patient. Examination findings that suggest a pelvic fracture include blood at the urethral meatus, a discrepancy in limb length, and a rotational deformity of the limb.[9]

Diagnosis and Initial Management

Hemodynamically unstable patients require resuscitation with large bore intravenous access and a 1:1:1 transfusion strategy (ie, equal transfusions of red blood cells, plasma, and platelets) while the appropriate next steps are being considered. Warming of the patient is also crucial given hypothermia may ensue. Hypothermia is one of the noted "lethal triad" of trauma leading to death, with acidosis and coagulopathy, the other 2 components. Recommended approaches for warming include warmed intravenous fluids, blankets, or mechanical warming devices.[4]

Laboratory evaluation is of limited utility in the initial evaluation of suspected abdominal vascular injuries, but it can provide a baseline for future monitoring and resuscitation efforts.

Radiography has little utility in the diagnosis of abdominal vascular injuries, with the one exception being a pelvis radiograph for the evaluation of an unstable pelvic fracture. The initial management of a hypotensive patient with suspected pelvic disruption includes the placement of a sheet or pelvic binder at the level of the greater trochanters of the femur to temporarily fixate the pelvis. Definitive management varies, but the most recent edition of Advanced Trauma Life Support notes that the presence of intraperitoneal blood is a key point in the management algorithm. Presence of intraperitoneal fluid dictates a laparotomy as the next step, whereas the absence dictates angiography and embolization by Interventional Radiology.[9]

The Focused Assessment with Sonography for Trauma (FAST) examination is a rapid tool in the identification of intraperitoneal fluid. There is controversy regarding its ability to detect vascular injury, with recent literature noting a sensitivity of 41%

when used in normotensive blunt trauma patients. This number increases if the operator is more skilled, with missed injury rates approaching 10%.[4]

Diagnostic peritoneal lavage (DPL) is another study that can be performed both rapidly and at the bedside. It has fallen out of favor more recently given the increased availability of less invasive diagnostic imaging modalities including ultrasound and computed tomography (CT). However, in hemodynamically normal patients who require abdominal evaluation in settings where FAST and CT cannot be readily performed, DPL may be a viable alternative.

CT, particularly CT angiography when there is a strong suspicion of a vascular injury, is more accurate at detecting vascular injuries and can also evaluate retroperitoneal and pelvic injuries. Because CT angiography typically requires transport from the primary resuscitation area, it should not be performed in those who are hemodynamically unstable.

Once a vascular injury has been determined, evaluation by a trauma surgeon is necessary. Both nonoperative and operative interventions are available for these patients depending on the clinical scenario.

Nontraumatic vascular abdominal emergencies include obstruction or rupture of the primary arteries and veins of the abdomen. Mortality is high and diagnosis is difficult, so the emergency provider must understand the pathology, clinical presentation, and management of these conditions. Nontraumatic vascular emergencies can be further subcategorized into bowel ischemia, both chronic and acute, and aortic and inferior vena cava pathology. In the following, the diagnosis and treatment of these conditions is discussed.

BOWEL ISCHEMIA

Bowel ischemia refers to insufficient oxygenation to meet demand to the small intestine (mesenteric ischemia) or large intestine (colonic ischemia) resulting in bowel necrosis.[5] One must understand the vascular anatomy to appreciate the underlying pathology. As discussed earlier, the SMA supplies blood flow to the entire small bowel except for the most proximal duodenum, which is perfused by the celiac artery. Both the SMA and the IMA perfuse the large intestine. The IMA is the primary blood supply for the colon from the splenic flexure to the rectum.[10] There is extensive collateral circulation to the bowel from the celiac artery, marginal artery of Drummond, and meandering mesenteric artery.[11] Two watershed areas most prone to ischemia are the splenic flexure and the rectosigmoid junction. The venous circulation mirrors the arterial circulation and drains into the portal system. Because of high collaterals, the bowel can withstand transient low blood flow states. However, prolonged ischemia leads to bowel necrosis from the inadequate perfusion to meet demand. The path to necrosis also has significant risk to the patient. When the bowel experiences low flow, vasoconstriction occurs, causing injury to the submucosa and mucosa, which affects the bowel's ability to protect against bacterial translocation precipitating sepsis,[12] and this triggers the inflammatory cascade worsening vasospasm and eventual necrosis of the bowel.[12] To understand the spectrum of bowel ischemia please see **Fig. 3**.

Clinical Presentation

Acute mesenteric ischemia accounts for 70% of cases of bowel ischemia and has a mortality rate of 60% to 80%.[13] Mesenteric ischemia affects women more than men and is more prevalent than appendicitis and abdominal aortic aneurysm (AAA) in the geriatric population.[14] The most common cause of acute mesenteric ischemia is

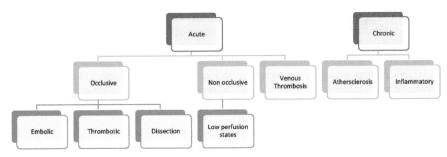

Fig. 3. Classification of bowel ischemia.

arterial embolism to the SMA accounting for 50% of the cases.[12] Other causes include thrombosis from underlying atherosclerosis (20%–35%) and dissection (<5%).[12] Risk factors include atherosclerosis and comorbidities that precipitate embolism such as atrial fibrillation, recent myocardial infarction, ventricular aneurysm, and prosthetic heart valves.[15] Delays in diagnosis and management accounts for the high mortality rate. Sudden onset of abdominal pain out of proportion to the physical examination in association with nausea and vomiting are the most common presenting symptom. Colonic ischemia has a similar pathophysiology as acute mesenteric ischemia but can be differentiated by the location and severity of pain. Colonic ischemia usually has less severe and more lateral abdominal pain and presents with hematochezia early in the clinical course.

Chronic arterial bowel ischemia is most commonly caused by underlying athero-sclerosis, which results in inappropriate blood flow to meet postprandial demands.[10] Chronic mesenteric ischemia affects women more than men and those older than 65 years with atherosclerosis risk factors.[10] Patients with vasculitis, fibromuscular dysplasia, malignancy, and radiation may also develop chronic mesenteric ischemia. Diagnosis is often difficult and requires a thorough clinical history to reveal postpran-dial pain, early satiety, and nausea and vomiting after eating. Anticipation of these symptoms can lead to a fear of eating with associated food restriction and weight loss.

Nonocclusive bowel ischemia is a result of systemic low flow states causing intes-tinal hypoperfusion. It accounts for one-third of cases of mesenteric ischemia and has a mortality rate of up to 80%.[16] It predominantly occurs at the watershed areas of the bowel described earlier. Risk factors include low cardiac output status, renal failure, liver failure, shock, abdominal compartment syndrome, vasopressor therapy, and other drugs that reduce splanchnic blood flow.

Mesenteric venous thrombosis in the bowel increases resistance to mesenteric blood flow, leading to arterial vasospasm and transmural bowel ischemia. It accounts for 6% of acute bowel ischemia with a mortality rate of 25%.[17] Inherited and acquired hypercoagulable states put a patient at risk for developing venous thrombosis.[13] Most acute venous thrombosis occurs in the superior mesenteric vein and less commonly in the portal or splenic vein.[13] Understanding those patients at risk for venous throm-bosis is critical, as the clinical examination and history is variable. The most sensitive clinical examination finding is abdominal pain out of proportion to the physical exam-ination. Patients may also describe subacute abdominal pain with anorexia, hemato-chezia, constipation, and nausea.

Diagnosis

One cannot emphasize enough the importance of clinical suspicion to minimize delays in diagnosis, as there are no reliable pathognomonic constellation of symptoms or clinically useful biomarkers to diagnose bowel ischemia.[12] Common laboratory abnormalities include elevated white blood cell counts with a left shift, azotemia, and lactate elevation. Clinical concern warrants appropriate imaging. Although ultrasound sensitivity nears 100%, it depends on operator skill, patient's body habitus, and the amount of arterial calcification.[14] A contrast-enhanced triphasic CT angiography is the gold standard and allows providers to appreciate sources of emboli, contributing intraabdominal pathology, and other potential diagnoses.[12,14,15] Concerning findings include pneumatosis intestinalis, portal vein gas, lack of bowel wall enhancement, mesenteric edema, and focal bowel wall edema.

Treatment

Big picture treatment of bowel ischemia is to reestablish perfusion to the bowel and prevent necrosis, but it ultimately varies on the underlying cause of the ischemia based on the classifications (see **Fig. 3**). In all cases, providers can improve outcomes by correctly managing the complications of low perfusion states in the bowel. In low flow states, inflammation increases the risk of bacterial translocation, resulting in sepsis. Broad spectrum antibiotics covering enteric gram negative and anaerobic bacteria improve clinical outcomes.[12] Fluid resuscitation to maintain euvolemia in the setting of sepsis or hypovolemia helps to optimize blood flow to the bowel and protect against further splanchnic vasoconstriction. If pressors are necessary after appropriate fluid resuscitation has been initiated, low-dose epinephrine or dopamine can improve cardiac function while minimizing effects on intestinal blood flow. Patients should be anticoagulated with heparin to prevent clot progression.[18] Finally, providers must be prepared to treat metabolic abnormalities including hyperkalemia, acute kidney injury, and metabolic acidosis.

Management of acute embolic mesenteric ischemia is rapidly changing with a progression toward a multidisciplinary team and the utilization of a hybrid endovascular and open procedure (**Fig. 4**) Traditionally, peritonitis suggested a need for laparotomy to assess the viability of the bowel.[19] In the setting of embolic mesenteric ischemia, a laparotomy would be combined with an open SMA embolectomy and resection of necrosed bowel. Mesenteric ischemia from thrombosis was classically managed

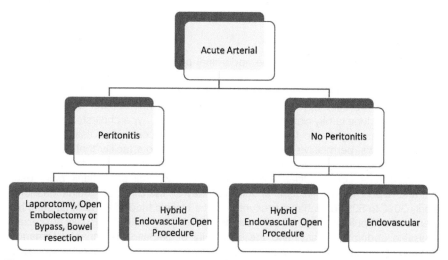

Fig. 4. Management algorithm for acute mesenteric ischemia.

with laparotomy and open bypass with an autologous vein graft to divert the critical atherosclerotic lesion.[19] However, there has been recent advancement in the use of endovascular procedures for the management of bowel ischemia. Endovascular procedures can be broadly broken into 3 categories: thrombolysis, pharmacomechanical thromboembolectomy, and angioplasty/stenting.[19] Thrombolysis involves catheter-directed lysis of an occlusion using lytic agents. This technique is most optimal for patients with no peritonitis and embolic occlusion. Pharmacomechanical thromboembolectomy uses devices that percutaneously break up and aspirate a thrombotic or embolic occlusion. Angioplasty with and without stenting has been used in chronic mesenteric ischemia in the past, but recent studies have shown success in the treatment of acute lesions as well. Despite the improvements in endovascular treatments, many patients will require laparotomy. Thus, many centers are transitioning to a hybrid endovascular and open approach for the management of bowel ischemia. This technique is specifically useful for thrombotic mesenteric ischemia where the SMA can be directly visualized, and a retrograde endovascular approach can treat the lesion, saving the patient a significant surgical bypass procedure. In addition, this combined approach allows the intervention on lesions not amendable to endovascular approach due to anatomy or ostial atherosclerosis.

Treatment of chronic mesenteric ischemia and venous thrombosis includes prompt anticoagulation management with a bolus and infusion of heparin. Chronic mesenteric ischemia treatment will also likely include endovascular angioplasty and stenting unless there is peritonitis at which point a hybrid approach can be considered.[18] Finally, in nonobstructive mesenteric ischemia the mainstay of treatment is to address the underlying cause with appropriate hemodynamic support.

Bowel ischemia is a challenging diagnosis with significant mortality and rapidly changing treatment protocol. Emergency medicine providers must consider intestinal ischemia in the differential of any older patient presenting with abdominal pain.

ABDOMINAL AORTIC PATHOLOGY

Abdominal aortic pathology includes aortic aneurysm with associated endovascular leak or rupture, aortic enteric fistula, and aortic occlusion. The high mortality associated with abdominal aortic pathology demands that emergency providers are well versed in the diagnosis and management of these conditions.

Abdominal Aortic Aneurysm

An AAA is pathologic dilation of the abdominal aorta of greater than 3 cm usually occurring below the renal arteries.[20] Progressive enlargement of the aorta places patients at risk for rupture, which carries a mortality rate of nearly 85%. This pathology affects men more than women, with the highest risk in those older than 65 years. Risk factors include family history, smoking, hypertension, hypercholesterolemia, prior vascular disease, systemic inflammation, and genetic connective tissue diseases. Timely diagnosis, permissive hypotension, and transfer to a facility that can perform endovascular or open repair are critical. AAA should be considered for any patient with appropriate comorbidities presenting with abdominal pain, flank pain, back pain, and hypotension. Clinicians should not relay on the clinical examination alone, as only 30% to 50% of patients present with the classic triad of abdominal pain, hypotension, and pulsatile mass. Body habitus may limit the ability to visually appreciate a pulsatile abdominal mass, and the sensitivity of palpation is variable. Bimanual palpation of supraumbilical area has a sensitivity of 61% for 3 to 3.9 cm aneurysms, 69% for those aneurysms 4 to 4.9 cm, and 82% for aneurysms 5 cm and larger.[21]

Diagnosis depends on clinical concern and demands immediate imaging. The gold-standard imaging is CT with intravenous contrast. CT has the advantage of defining the anatomy of the aorta and the location of the rupture, which is critical to identify if a patient is amendable to endovascular repair.[21] Also, it has improved sensitivity of identifying suprarenal aneurysms. Although CT scan remains the diagnostic imaging of choice for surgical planning, obtaining a CT scan depends on patient stability and can delay transfer to a treatment facility. With the improved skill of emergency physicians, point-of-care ultrasound (POCUS) is becoming a reliable means of early diagnosis to guide immediate treatment. ED POCUS has a sensitivity of 99% for identifying aneurysm but is less consistent in its ability to identify rupture.[22] The difficulty in identifying rupture with ultrasound is likely attributable to the fact that most of the AAAs rupture into the retroperitoneal space, making visualization difficult.[22]

Once a diagnosis of AAA is made, the Society for Vascular Surgery recommends repair within 90 minutes of presentation. Endovascular repair requires specific anatomic criteria, which are usually defined through CT imaging. Thus, the emergency provider must optimize hemodynamic status while awaiting ultimate treatment considerations. Current literature supports permissive hypotension to maintain mental status and systolic blood pressure of 70 to 100 mm Hg.[20] Permissive hypotension promotes clot stability through minimizing rapid increases in systolic blood pressure that can lead to clot disruption and associated progression of hemorrhagic shock.[20] If resuscitation is necessary emphasis should be placed on packed red blood cells. Avoiding fluid resuscitation helps limits dilution of clotting factors, platelets, and fibrinogen.[23] Abdominal aortic aneurysm rupture is a high mortality condition that can easily be missed. The emergency provider must be able to quickly diagnose and provide goal-oriented hemodynamic management to improve outcomes.

Complications of abdominal aortic aneurysm repair

It is critical for emergency providers to understand the workup and treatment of endograft complications, which occurs in 30% of cases.[20] Complications include endograft leak, angulation, kinking, migration, or thrombosis. Endoleak is the most prevalent complication that results in the leakage of blood between the graft and the aneurysm sac, which puts patients at risk of rerupture. (Clancy, 2019) Symptoms include back or abdominal pain, but most are asymptomatic. CT angiography is the most sensitive means of evaluation. The management of an endograft leak is identical to AAA rupture including permissive hypotension and endovascular repair. Patients who have undergone endovascular aortic repair or open aortic repair are at risk of graft infection. Any patient with an aortic graft presenting with sepsis of unknown cause or new pseudoaneurysm near the aortic graft should be treated as a presumed graft infection.[24] There is no established diagnostic gold standard for graft infection, and imaging results can be subtle. CT findings that suggest graft infection include perigraft fluid more than 3 months postprocedure or perigraft gas more than 7 weeks postprocedure.[24] Emergency department management should include administration of broad-spectrum antibiotics and emergent vascular surgery consultation for operative intervention.

The most feared complication of aortic aneurysm repair is the development of an aortoenteric fistula (AEF). Although AEF can occur due to pathologies of a native aorta, most of the AEF occur in the setting of previous aortic surgery. AEF usually develops within 2 weeks of surgery but can develop up to 8 years postsurgery. Even if symptoms are transient, patients after aortic surgery who present with melena, hematochezia, or syncope should be presumed to have AEF. The "herald bleed" is a well-documented phenomenon in AEF where a small bleed occurs that is temporarily sealed off through thrombus formation. However, if the "herald bleed" is not recognized, diagnosed, and treated emergently, the temporary clot can destabilize, leading to exsanguination.[25]

In suspected AEF, CT angiography is the gold standard with a sensitivity of 94% and specificity of 85%.[26] Findings include ectopic gas within or near the aorta, focal bowel wall thickening, perigraft inflammation, or extravasation of contrast material into the bowel lumen.[26] A high index of suspicion is essential in achieving a timely diagnosis and intervention at the time of the "herald bleed." Management for both primary and secondary AEF include broad spectrum antibiotics, reversal of anticoagulation, massive transfusion, and involvement of vascular surgery to progress to open or endovascular operative repair.[27]

Aortic Occlusion

Although rare, aortic occlusion is a life-threatening condition that cannot be overlooked. The most common location for aortic occlusion is at the bifurcation of the aorta. In situ thrombosis in an already atherosclerotic aorta accounts for 64% of cases (Grip O, 2019). Other causes include migration of a large saddle embolus from the proximal aorta or heart and occlusion of aortic grafts or stents. Those at risk for the development of aortic occlusion are patients with atherosclerosis, dysrhythmias, smoking, hypercoagulable states, and previous surgical intervention. Symptoms depend on the level of the occlusion but commonly include signs of acute limb ischemia (pallor, pulselessness, pain, paresthesia), neurologic deficits (paralysis, pain, numbness), and abdominal pain. CT angiography is the best modality for direct anatomic visualization of the occlusion and concomitant atherosclerosis. Treatment depends on the underlying cause of the occlusion. Management of in situ thrombosis, now the most common cause, involves open bypass surgery. Graft thrombosis or embolectomy are usually treated with endovascular interventions including thromboembolectomy or catheter-directed thrombolysis (Grip O, 2019).

The high morbidity and mortality of abdominal aortic pathology can be minimized by maintaining a high index of suspicion and expeditiously arranging transfer to a facility capable of open or endovascular management.

Nontraumatic vascular abdominal emergencies are subtle in presentation but carry a high mortality. Emergency medicine providers must consider intestinal ischemia in the differential of any older patient presenting with abdominal pain. Although acute bowel ischemia can be both occlusive and nonocclusive; embolic occlusive is the most common and current treatments focus on a hybrid multidisciplinary team approach. Abdominal aortic aneurysm rupture is a catastrophic condition that requires permissive hypotension and repair within 90 minutes. Complications from AAA repair are common and critical to diagnose and manage appropriately.

CLINICS CARE POINTS

- The lack of abdominal tenderness on examination does not rule out an intraabdominal vascular injury.
- Instability of the pelvic ring should be considered in those with blunt trauma with possible pelvic fractures. If hypotensive, the initial management includes the placement of a sheet or pelvic binder at the level of the greater trochanters of the femur to temporarily fixate the pelvis.
- In the elderly population, abdominal pain out of proportion warrants CT angiography to rule out acute mesenteric ischemia.

- Treatment of mesenteric ischemia involves identifying the cause and managing complications.
  - Broad spectrum antibiotics
  - Fluid resuscitation to a euvolemic state
  - Anticipate metabolic derangement: hyperkalemia, acute kidney injury, acidosis
- For acute occlusive mesenteric ischemia
  - Start anticoagulation
  - Manage complications as mentioned earlier
  - Transfer to a facility that can coordinate hybrid endovascular and open surgical management
- AAA
  - Manual palpation has a low sensitivity
  - POCUS depends on body habitus and operator skill
  - CT with intravenous contrast is the gold standard
  - Permissive hypotension with systolic blood pressures from 70 to 100 mm Hg improves outcomes
  - Packed red blood cells to maintain systolic blood pressure and mental status
  - Repair within 90 minutes with endovascular or open procedure

DISCLOSURE

The authors have no commercial or financial disclosures.

REFERENCES

1. Lewiss RE, Egan DJ, Shreves A. Vascular abdominal emergencies. Emerg Med Clin North Am 2011;29(2):253–72, viii.
2. Kobayashi L, costantini T, Hamel M, et al. Abdominal vascular trauma. Trauma Surg Acute Care Open 2016;1:1–7.
3. Dua AD, Holcomb JB, Burgess AR, et al. Clinical review of vascular trauma. Springer Publishing; 2013.
4. Kobayashi L, Coimbra R, Goes AMO Jr, et al. American Association for the Surgery of Trauma-World Society of Emergency Surgery guidelines on diagnosis and management of abdominal vascular injuries. J Trauma Acute Care Surg 2020; 89(6):1197–211.
5. Selim M, Alnaimi MI, Alsadah ZY, et al. Different treatment modality in the management of acute mesenteric ischemia. Cureus 2021;13(1):e12490.
6. Lamb CM, Garner JP. Selective non-operative management of civilian gunshot wounds to the abdomen: a systematic review of the evidence. Injury 2014; 45(4):659–66.
7. Shanmuganathan K, Mirvis SE, Chiu WC, et al. Penetrating torso trauma: triple-contrast helical CT in peritoneal violation and organ injury–a prospective study in 200 patients. Radiology 2004;231(3):775–84.
8. Nishijima DK, Simel DL, Wisner DH, et al. Does this adult patient have a blunt intra-abdominal injury? Jama 2012;307(14):1517–27.
9. Surgeons AACo. ATLS advanced trauma life support 10th edition student course manual. 10th edition 2018.
10. Huber TS, Björck M, Chandra A, et al. Chronic mesenteric ischemia: clinical practice guidelines from the Society for Vascular Surgery. J Vasc Surg 2021;73(1s): 87s–115s.
11. Walker TG. Meseteric vasculatrure and collateral pathways. Semin Intervent Radiol 2009;26(3):167–74.

12. Clair DG, Beach JM. Mesenteric ischemia. N Engl J Med 2016;374(10):959–68.
13. Cruz RJ Jr, Garrido AG, Ribeiro CM, et al. Regional blood flow distribution and oxygen metabolism during mesenteric ischemia and congestion. J Surg Res 2010;161(1):54–61.
14. Reintam Blaser A, Preiser JC, Fruhwald S, et al. Gastrointestinal dysfunction in the critically ill: a systematic scoping review and research agenda proposed by the section of metabolism, endocrinology and nutrition of the European Society of Intensive Care Medicine. Crit Care 2020;24(1):224.
15. Prichayudh S, Rassamee P, Sriussadaporn S, et al. Abdominal vascular injuries: blunt vs. penetrating. Injury 2019;50(1):137–41.
16. Al-Diery H, Phillips A, Evennett N, et al. The pathogenesis of nonocclusive mesenteric ischemia: implications for research and clinical practice. J Intensive Care Med 2019;34(10):771–81.
17. Blumberg SN, Maldonado TS. Mesenteric venous thrombosis. J Vasc Surg Venous Lymphat Disord 2016;4(4):501–7.
18. Luther B, Mamopoulos A, Lehmann C, et al. The ongoing challenge of acute mesenteric ischemia. Clin Ther Rev 2018;34:217–23.
19. Prakash VS, Marin M, Faries PL. Acute and chronic ischemic disorders of the small bowel. Curr Gastroenterol Rep 2019;21(6):27.
20. Meyermann KCF. Treatment of abdominal aortic pathology. Cardiol Clin 2017;35: 431–9.
21. Sakalihasan N, Limet R, Defawe OD. Abdominal aortic aneurysm. Lancet 2005; 365(9470):1577–89.
22. Diaz O, Eilbert W. Ruptured abdominal aortic aneurysm identified on point-of-care ultrasound in the emergency department. Int J Emerg Med 2020;13(1):25.
23. Moreno DH, Cacione DG, Baptista-Silva JC. Controlled hypotension versus normotensive resuscitation strategy for people with ruptured abdominal aortic aneurysm. Cochrane Database Syst Rev 2018;6(6):Cd011664.
24. Lyons OT, Baguneid M, Barwick TD, et al. Diagnosis of aortic graft infection: a case definition by the management of aortic graft infection collaboration (MAGIC). Eur J Vasc Endovasc Surg 2016;52(6):758–63.
25. Gordon AC, Agarwal M. Primary aorto-enteric fistula. Int J Surg Case Rep 2016; 19:60–2.
26. Hughes FM, Kvanagh D, Barry M, et al. Aortoeneteric fistula: a diagnostic dilemma. Abdom Imaging 2007;32:398–402.
27. Dorosh J, Lin JC. Aortoenterofistula. In: StatPearls. StatPearls Publishing LLC; 2021.

Postprocedural Gastrointestinal Emergencies

Brian K. Parker, MD[a], Sara Manning, MD[b],*

KEYWORDS

- Complications • Laparoscopy • Endoscopy • Bariatric surgery
- Interventional radiology • Mesh

KEY POINTS

- Postprocedural complications can present hours to years after their index procedure.
- Complications may be anatomic, mechanical, infectious, or metabolic in nature.
- A thorough history of prior surgeries and procedures is an important component of the emergency department evaluation of abdominal pain.

INTRODUCTION

The last 50 years have seen incredible advancements in diagnostic and therapeutic procedures for a wide array of conditions. As procedural safety measures continue to improve, many procedures from endoscopy to general surgery have transitioned to the ambulatory setting. In 2010, more than 48 million procedures, both surgical and nonsurgical, were performed at ambulatory centers in the United States.[1] This trend is of particular interest to the emergency physician, as patients who develop complications often present to an emergency department for evaluation and treatment. Here the authors examine a collection of procedures notable for their frequent utilization and unique complication profiles including laparoscopic surgery, bariatric surgery, endoscopic procedures, interventional radiology procedures, and hernia repairs with implantable mesh.

Laparoscopic Procedures

General complications of laparoscopy

Laparoscopy, in and of itself, can lead to a variety of complications. Laparoscopic surgery of the abdominal or pelvic organs requires insufflation of the peritoneal space with gas, most typically carbon dioxide. Insufflation can result in abdominal

[a] Department of Emergency Medicine, University of Texas Health San Antonio, 7703 Floyd Curl Drive, MC 7736, San Antonio, TX 78229, USA; [b] Department of Emergency Medicine, Indiana University School of Medicine, 720 Eskenazi Avenue | FOB 3rd Floor, Indianapolis, IN 46202, USA
* Corresponding author.
E-mail address: smanning4@iuhealth.org

Emerg Med Clin N Am 39 (2021) 781–794
https://doi.org/10.1016/j.emc.2021.07.008
0733-8627/21/© 2021 Elsevier Inc. All rights reserved.

discomfort. There is also potential risk of gas tracking through the anatomic hiatus of the diaphragm, resulting in subcutaneous emphysema, pneumomediastinum, or pneumothorax, with additional risk of tension physiology.[2]

Gas embolism is a rare but potentially catastrophic insufflation-associated complication. Gas embolism can occur due to inadvertent placement of the insufflating needle into a vascular or parenchymal structure or as a result of vascular injury. Gas embolization can occur at the time of initial insufflation or at any point intraoperatively. Presentation varies with the amount, nature, and distribution (venous vs arterial) of embolized gas. Small, venous emboli are frequently observed and are rarely symptomatic.[3] Large venous emboli, emboli of non-CO2 gases and arterial emboli can cause acute neurologic deficits, organ infarction, cardiovascular collapse, and death.[3,4] As such, patients who suffer severe intraoperative gas embolism in an ambulatory surgical setting would require immediate transfer to an emergency department. Patients may demonstrate hypotension, dyspnea, cyanosis, and a sloshing, mill-wheel murmur.[4] Intraoperative use of non-CO2 gases (argon, helium, and so forth) and inadequate flushing of air from insufflating lines may result in emboli of less water-soluble gases, complicating treatment.[5–7] If suspected, the patient should be oxygenated with 100% Fio_2 and placed in a left lateral decubitus position in Trendelenburg ("Durant position") in attempts to trap gas in the ventricles and prevent further embolization. Gas emboli may be observed via point-of-care ultrasound (US).[3,5] If gas is observed in the right chambers, gas may be aspirated via a central line.[5,6] Hyperbaric oxygen therapy can be beneficial.[5,6]

Improvements in surgical site infections contributed to the increase in popularity of laparoscopy; however, port-site infections (PSI) remain relatively common.[8] The incidence of PSI varies with presence of infectious pathogens in the target organ, operative technique, and patient comorbidities.[9,10] PSI are most commonly observed in umbilical ports and are often attributed to wound contamination by umbilical flora, although this is controversial.[10,11] Extraction of an inflamed or infected organ through a port site, use of an extraction bag, and patient factors such as diabetes, obesity, and smoking may also increase risk of PSI.[8,9,12] Although abdominal wall emphysema is common, increased pain, erythema, and purulent drainage suggest PSI. Most port-site infections are superficial and resolve with oral antibiotics but necrotizing soft tissue infections have been reported.[13]

Although of lesser clinical significance, postoperative shoulder pain is among the most commonly observed complications of laparoscopic surgery, occurring in as many as 75% of patients.[14] Attributed to diaphragmatic irritation by retained gas and distention-induced neuropraxia of the phrenic nerve, postoperative shoulder pain is a benign condition that may be observed for several days postoperatively, typically improving within 24 to 72 hours.[15,16] Worsening of pain after initial improvement or associated vital sign abnormalities are atypical and should prompt further evaluation. Treatment with nonsteroidal antiinflammatory drugs and glucocorticoids is recommended.[16]

Cholecystectomy

Laparoscopic cholecystectomy is among the most common general surgical procedures performed in the United States.[1] The 30-day complication rate of cholecystectomy is approximately 10%, but clinically significant complications are rare.[17] The most common early complications include infection (2%) and intestinal disorders including ileus and obstruction (1.9%).[17]

The most feared complication of laparoscopic cholecystectomy is bile duct injury (BDI). Through advancements in instrumentation and technique, the increased risk of BDI observed in the early days of laparoscopy has decreased significantly.[17,18] BDIs currently complicate approximately 0.23% of laparoscopic cholecystectomies.[17] The Hannover Classification System describes 5 injury patterns of biliary leaks or obstructions with variable clinical significance based on anatomic location (**Table 1**).[19] BDI with or without associated vascular injury may develop secondary to a myriad of causes, including misidentification of anatomic structures, malpositioned clips, or injury from cautery or dissection (**Fig. 1**).[2,19] Most BDIs are identified at the index operation, but as many as 28% may be missed with greater than 14% presenting more than a month after the procedure.[17] Common symptoms at presentation include right upper quadrant pain, nausea, vomiting, fever, and jaundice.[2] The imaging modality of choice for suspected BDI is computed tomography (CT) of the abdomen and pelvis with contrast, although MRI and US may also be diagnostic.[20] Many BDIs will require drainage through either endoscopic or percutaneous techniques with the remainder requiring operative intervention.[17,21] Broad-spectrum antibiotics including coverage for methicillin-resistant *Staphylococcus aureus* (MRSA) and enteric pathogens is recommended.[22]

Appendicitis

Appendicitis is the most common surgical emergency world-wide.[8] More than 225,000 laparoscopic appendectomies are attempted each year in the United States with a conversion rate of approximately 6.3%.[23] Laparoscopic approaches are associated with shorter hospital length of stay, wound infection, and return to normal activity but an increased risk of intraabdominal abscess (1.2% in open resection vs 2% in

Table 1		
Hannover classification of bile duct injuries		
Hannover Classification	**Injury**	**Subgroup**
A	Peripheral bile leak	• A1: cystic duct leak • A2: gallbladder bed
B	Stenosis of the main bile duct without injury (may include vascular injury)	• B1: incomplete • B2: complete
C	Tangential injury of the bile duct	• C1: punctiform lesion <5 mm • C2: 5 mm lesion below hepatic bifurcation • C3: 5 mm lesion at the hepatic bifurcation • C4: 5 mm lesion above the hepatic bifurcation
D	Transection of the bile duct	• D1: without defect below the hepatic bifurcation • D2: with defect below the hepatic bifurcation • D3: at the hepatic bifurcation with or without defect • D4: above the hepatic bifurcation with or without defect
E	Bile duct strictures	• E1: short, circular <5 mm, CHD or CBD • E2: longitudinal CBD >5 mm • E3: stricture at hepatic bifurcation • E4: right hepatic or segmental bile ducts

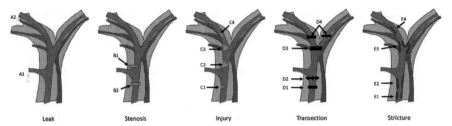

Fig. 1. Hannover classification of bile duct injuries: A1—cystic duct leak, A2—leak in gallbladder bed; B1—incomplete stenosis, B2—complete stenosis; C1—punctate lesion <5 mm, C2—>5 mm lesion below the bifurcation, C3—>5 mm lesion at the bifurcation, C4—>5 mm lesion above the bifurcation, D1—transection below the bifurcation without defect, D2—transection below the bifurcation with defect, D3—transection at the bifurcation with or without defect, D4—transection above the bifurcation with or without defect; E1—short segment (<5 mm) stricture below the bifurcation, E2—long (>5 mm)segment stricture below the bifurcation, E3—stricture at the bifurcation, E4—stricture of right main or segmental bile duct.

laparoscopic).[24] Greater than 90% of postappendectomy abscesses are observed in those with gangrenous or perforated appendicitis.[25] Diagnosis can be confirmed with contrasted CT or US.[25,26] Treatment varies widely with size of the abscess and clinical presentation of the patient and can include watchful waiting, intravenous antibiotics, percutaneous drainage, or operative drainage.[25]

Stump appendicitis is a rare late complication of appendectomy characterized by interval reinflammation of residual appendiceal tissue. Larger residual stumps are a risk factor, but stump appendicitis has been observed in stumps as short as 5 mm.[27] The most common presenting symptoms include right lower quadrant or generalized abdominal pain and fever.[27] Both US and CT can be diagnostic, and operative resection is the treatment of choice.[27]

Postbariatric Surgery

The incidence of obesity has been steadily increasing over the past 50 years, and, as of 2016, 40% of adults in the United States meet the definition of obese.[28] Likewise, there has been a concurrent increase in the number of metabolic and bariatric surgeries, peaking at 252,000 in 2017.[29] The most common of these procedures performed in the United States is the sleeve gastrectomy, in which a portion of the greater curvature of the stomach is removed to reduce the overall size of the stomach. The biliopancreatic diversion with duodenal switch is a procedure that is growing in popularity but is usually restricted to those with body mass index greater than 50 due to the higher risk of complications.[30] Endoscopic weight loss procedures are also growing in popularity; gastric balloon insertion is a popular procedure in which a fluid- or gas-filled device is used to occupy a large portion of the stomach.[31] Older, less common procedures that are still performed in some places in the world and were previously popular include roux-en-Y gastric bypass (RYGBP), biliopancreatic diversion, gastric banding, and stomach folding. Although the overall complication rate of all these procedures is low, 6% of those complications require a second operative procedure.[32] The most common complications can include internal hernias, anastomotic leak, strictures, and malabsorptive disorders.

Internal hernia

An internal hernia occurs when a loop of bowel passes through a mesenteric defect or at an anastomosis. Internal hernias can become incarcerated or strangulated causing significant pain. They can also act as a transition point, leading to small bowel obstruction.[33] Patients who have undergone RYGBP are at particular risk for internal hernia due to multiple mesenteric defects created during the course of the procedure. In postbariatric surgery patients, up to 50% of all small bowel obstructions are attributed to internal hernias, and traditional nasogastric tube placement for decompression as well as conservative management is more likely to fail. In early postop RYGBP patients, dilation of the gastric remnant can lead to perforation and high mortality.[34]

Anastomotic leak and marginal ulcer

The most common cause of early death in postoperative bariatric surgery patients is an anastomotic leak.[35] This leak most commonly occurs in the first 10 days following the procedure and can occur in up to 6% of post-RYGBP patients.[36] These patients do not present with classic peritoneal signs but most commonly present with tachycardia greater than 120 beats per minute.[37] Physical examination findings are not reliable and early surgical consultation as well as early contrasted CT imaging are essential for making the diagnosis.

Marginal ulcers can occur in up to 16% of gastric bypass procedures.[38] There are no identified risk factors, and the cause of the ulceration is not well established, although increased acidity is one of the proposed mechanisms.[39] The patient's presentation can vary from essentially asymptomatic to severe postprandial pain and rarely perforation.[40] Marginal ulcers generally will occur within the first month of surgery and rarely after 1 year postop.[40,41] Early referral to endoscopy can assist in the diagnosis, and initiation of a proton pump inhibitor may help reduce progression of the disease.[41]

Postbariatric surgery gastrointestinal hemorrhage can occur at any time in the postoperative course and has been reported decades after the procedure.[42,43] Early postoperative bleeding is associated with longer hospital stays and a mortality of 3.8% versus less than 1% for those without early bleeding.[42] In gastric bypass patients, 15% will develop an ulcer in the first 3 months after surgery.[35] Late GI bleeds, those more than 1 year postsurgery, are very strongly associated with bleeding marginal ulceration of the gastrojejunostomy, with 0.6% to 12% of post-RYGBP patients demonstrating marginal ulcers on routine endoscopy.[43] Depending on the type of surgery, routine endoscopic techniques may be unable to reach the source of bleeding due to altered anatomy.[35]

Metabolic/electrolyte

Nutritional abnormalities are rare complications in the patients who receive restrictive methods of weight loss surgery (eg, lap band, sleeve gastrectomy, intragastric balloons) but are more common in the malabsorptive surgeries.[32] These abnormalities rarely present as an emergency condition but rather are identified during the patient's evaluation. The most common cause of these abnormalities is nonadherence to the recommended diet, including alcohol abuse.[44] Iron deficiency and B12 deficiency anemia are the most common causes of nutritional anemias in these patients.[35] In addition, vitamin D, thiamine, and folate can be deficient, although these are less common in the United States due to widespread availability of enriched foods.[44] Longstanding folate or thiamine deficiencies can occur, and there have been reports of peripheral neuropathy and Wernicke encephalopathy.[35]

Postendoscopy

More than 6 million outpatient endoscopies are performed in the United States each year, including upper endoscopy and colonoscopy.[1] Mild, transient abdominal pain and bloating are common but serious adverse events remain rare.[45,46] Perforation and significant bleeding are the most common of these serious adverse events and are noted in 0.5/1000 and 2.6/1000 colonoscopies, respectively.[46] Death due to colonoscopy complication is exceptionally rare (0.003%). However, given the frequency with which these procedures are performed, colonoscopies are associated with hundreds of deaths each year in the United States. Adverse event rates are higher for therapeutic endoscopies as opposed to screening procedures, likely due to underlying abnormal mucosa.[46] Perforation and bleeding may present hours to days following the procedure.

Perforation

Perforation may occur during any endoscopic procedure. Perforation rates from upper endoscopy range widely from 1/2500 to 1/11,000.[47,48] In a large pooled analysis of nearly 2 million colonoscopies, the perforation rate was estimated at 0.5/1000 procedures. Polypectomy was associated with an increased perforation rate at 0.8/1000 cases with polypectomy versus 0.4/1000 without polypectomy.[46] Most colonic perforations occur in the sigmoid colon.[49] Proposed mechanisms for perforation include stretch and shearing injuries, overinsufflation with resultant barotrauma, and complications of therapeutic manipulation, including thermal injury or blind passage of an instrument.[45] Abnormal underlying mucosa can increase the risk of perforation in all of these mechanisms.

Both esophageal and colonic perforations may be missed during the endoscopic procedure. More than half of colonic perforations have a delayed presentation, with some patients presenting weeks after their procedure.[49]

Delayed symptoms of esophageal perforation include fever, retrosternal chest pain, dyspnea, crepitus, and sepsis. The mortality rate of esophageal perforation remains as high as 18%.[50] Contrast esophagram using water-soluble contrast is favored for stable patients versus CT for those who are unstable.[50,51] Early identification and treatment of esophageal perforation can reduce morbidity and mortality.[51]

Patients with iatrogenic colonic perforation may describe persistent and increasing abdominal pain that becomes generalized, absence of flatus, and worsening abdominal distention. Abdominal tenderness with peritoneal signs can be observed on examination. Plain radiography of the chest or abdomen can demonstrate free air in 88% of cases; however CT with contrast can provide more diagnostic detail regarding location and severity of the injury.[49]

Esophageal and colonic perforations require emergent treatment with broad spectrum antibiotics and often require procedural or operative intervention.[49–51] Some perforations may be successfully treated with nonoperative approaches including observation with antimicrobials and bowel rest, endoscopic stenting or repair, and percutaneous drainage of abscesses.[45,51]

Bleeding

Bleeding is an important complication of endoscopy, particularly colonoscopy. In their review of nearly 2 million colonoscopies, Reumkens and colleagues found an overall bleeding rate of 0.26%, with higher rates observed in patients undergoing therapeutic colonoscopy including those performed in symptomatic patients (1.3%) and procedures with polypectomies (0.98%).[46] Significant bleeding after upper endoscopy is rare and is often attributed to lacerations and tears along the gastroesophageal junction.[45] Postpolypectomy bleeding is commonly observed in a delayed presentation, with most cases presenting several days after the procedure.[52] Risk factors for bleeding after colonoscopy include patient and procedural factors, most notably early resumption of anticoagulation within a week of the procedure and polyp size. For every 1 mm increase in polyp diameter, the risk of hemorrhage has been noted to increase by 9%.[52] Delayed bleeding is thought to be secondary to thermocoagulation-induced ulceration at the polypectomy site.[45]

Patients can present with typical symptoms of gastrointestinal hemorrhage including hematochezia, melena, and symptomatic anemia. Nearly half of all postpolypectomy hemorrhage patients will require transfusion.[52] Although postpolypectomy hemorrhage may resolve spontaneously, many will require a repeat colonoscopy. Those with continued hemorrhage not corrected by endoscopic techniques may require angiography with embolization or operative intervention.

Pancreatitis

Pancreatitis is the most common complication of endoscopic retrograde cholangiopancreatography (ERCP), with an estimated incidence of nearly 9.7%.[53,54] Post-ERCP pancreatitis (PEP) has a wide range of severity with most patients developing only mild symptoms. However, cases can lead to critical illness and death with an overall mortality rate of 0.7%.

The pathogenesis of PEP remains unclear. Cytokine release due to pancreatic acinar cell injury is thought to play a significant role.[53] Acinar cell injury may occur through a variety of mechanisms including mechanical injury from cannulation trauma or tissue manipulation, contrast-associated injuries including hydrostatic and chemical injury, and enzymatic and microbiological factors.[55] PEP risk factors include sphincter of Oddi dysfunction, female gender, prior history of pancreatitis as well as procedure-related risk factors including prolonged duration of cannulation attempts, more than one passage of the pancreatic guidewire and pancreatic injection.[56]

Pancreatic injury due to ERCP progresses quickly with measurable increases in lipase and amylase in less than 2 hours, frequently preceding the development of nausea and abdominal pain.[57] In the absence of PEP, amylase and lipase values peak at 90 minutes to 4 hours postprocedure and fall to normal at 48 hours.[55] C-reactive protein and interleukin-6 may be predictive of PEP severity.[58] A diagnostic approach using clinical assessment and laboratory studies is generally recommended, as history and physical examination alone demonstrate poor sensitivity for PEP. Supportive care emphasizing early hydration remains the mainstay of treatment of PEP. Antibiotics may be of benefit in patients with infected necrotizing pancreatitis; however, the routine use of prophylactic antibiotics even in severe pancreatitis is not recommended.[59]

Complications with Mesh and Hernia Repairs

Hernia repairs, including ventral hernia repair, are among the most common surgical procedures performed in the United States. Most are repaired with implantable mesh, as the addition of mesh decreases the incidence of recurrence.[60] Other common types of hernia repairs include incisional hernias, umbilical and epigastric hernias, and parastomal hernias. The 2 most feared complications associated with mesh hernia repairs are mesh failure and postplacement infection.

Mesh failure

There are several reasons that mesh placement could be considered a failure and require removal including recurrence of the hernia, pain, numbness, neuralgia, and mesh-related reaction.[61] Approximately 13% of mesh placements ultimately require removal, primarily due to the development of chronic pain.[61] In one study, the recurrence rate of hernias was 16.1%, with open hernia repairs failing more often than laparoscopic. However, most studies cite a much lower 1% failure rate.[62–64] The Ventral Hernia Outcomes Collaborative released a consensus statement regarding modifiable risk factors for mesh failure, highlighting morbid obesity and tobacco use.[65] Mesh placed in the pelvis was most commonly found to cause chronic pain requiring removal, whereas the mesh placed in the abdomen was more commonly removed due to infection.[61]

Women who have mesh placed to repair inguinal/pelvic hernias are much more likely to have chronic pain from the mesh insertion. Women have proportionally more inner-vation of pain receptors in the region, which is most likely the cause of this increase in incidence of chronic pain.[66] Mesh-related reactions are significantly more likely to be a cause of mesh removal in the groin than in the abdomen.[61] A recently described vari-ation of mesh failure is that of a "meshoma," a folding or balling up of the mesh causing compression of the surrounding tissue with associated chronic pain. Meshomas may present as hernia recurrence as well.[15,61] In pelvic repairs, meshomas have been found to cause worse nerve entrapment requiring neurectomy.[61] Most of these indica-tions for hernia mesh repair can be performed as an outpatient, unless a severe complication, such as incarceration, uncontrolled pain, or infection, occurs.[60]

Infection

It is thought that the rates of postsurgical infection performed with mesh are the same as those performed without mesh closure.[64] Any patient with a recent hernia repair presenting with abdominal pain, fever, or other infectious symptoms should be eval-uated for postoperative infection, including infected mesh. Although the immediate postoperative period is the most common time for mesh-related infections to develop, it has been reported to occur any time between 2 weeks to greater than 3 years following the initial procedure.[64] It is not uncommon for an immediate postop patient to have a residual seroma, which is not an infectious process, but any attempt by the emergency physician to aspirate it or perform a paracentesis near the area may inoc-ulate the fluid with bacteria.[64] It is classically taught that any infected meshes need to be removed, but there is some literature to support determining the need for reopera-tion based on the type of mesh used.[67]

Historically, infected inguinal mesh devices were found to grow out gram-positive bacteria, most commonly *S aureus*, with other cultures growing group B streptococci and *Peptostreptococcus*.[68] Given the growing prevalence of MRSA, any patient pre-senting with infected mesh should be given antibiotics with appropriate coverage based on a local antibiogram. Although there is scant data regarding anaerobic bac-teria infections, anaerobic coverage should also be initiated in a systemically ill patient. If the patient is too ill to be taken to the operating room for mesh removal, then a percu-taneous drain should be placed, as these deeper infections respond poorly to antibi-otics without source control.[69]

Types of parenteral feeding tubes and associated complications

There are 3 types of parenteral feeding tubes that are commonly placed: gastrostomy tubes (g-tubes), jejunal tubes (j-tubes), and gastrojejunal tubes (GJ-tubes).[70] G-tubes terminate in the stomach, a j-tube terminates in the proximal small bowel, and a GJ-tube has multiple ports, one of which terminates in the stomach and a second that ter-minates in the proximal small bowel. These types of tubes can be placed via an open surgical procedure, via an interventional radiology procedure or more commonly percutaneously.[71] There is no difference in mortality or morbidity associated with nonsurgical placements, and bedside percutaneous placement is becoming more common in patients in intensive care unit.[72]

Emergency department–specific postprocedural complications that are unique to parenteral feeding tube placement include buried bumper syndrome, gastric outlet obstruction, percutaneous endoscopic gastronomy (PEG) site herniation, and tube dislodgement.[70–73] Buried bumper syndrome is a rare complication, in which the internal bolster migrates out of the stomach toward the skin due to overtightening of the external bolster.[74] This migration causes pain and can lead to bleeding, perforation, abscess development, or peritonitis.[75] Occasionally, the bumper can be palpated in the subcutaneous tissue, but the diagnosis is confirmed via endoscopy.[71] In a similar manner, the distal portion of the g-tube can migrate toward the pylorus, causing an obstruction of the outlet, leading to high residuals feeds, crampy abdominal pain, and increasing risk for aspiration or vomiting. This generally occurs when the external bolster is loosened or lost. An abdominal radiograph will reveal mispositioning of the g-tube; gentle traction can safely reposition the tube and the bolster can then be tightened.[73]

PEG site herniation is an incredibly rare complication where the stomach can herniate through the stoma, leaking gastric contents on the skin, causing severe ulceration[76,77]; this can be diagnosed by CT scan of the abdomen and requires surgical consultation for operative repair.

Tube dislodgement is one of the most common presentations for parenteral feeding tube complications. Up to 4% of all PEG tube patients inadvertently remove their feeding tube at some point during its use.[71] The 2 most important factors for the emergency physician to consider are the tube type and the duration that it has been in place. J-tubes and GJ-tubes cannot be reinserted blindly and instead require interventional radiology or endoscopic replacement. These patients may require admission to for these procedures or parenteral administration of critical medications and hydration. Generally, 1 month after placement, the stomach has adhered to the abdominal wall and the tract is mature. If the tract is immature, there is a risk that the stomach has separated from the abdominal wall, and blind reinsertion is contraindicated. If a g-tube is dislodged within 1 month of placement, intravenous antibiotics should be initiated, the patient should be made NPO, and admitted to the hospital for subsequent replacement.[73]

Mature tracts begin to close within 1 day of tube dislodgement; therefore blind reinsertion is preferred. A new similar sized g-tube should be inserted through the tract, then the balloon inflated. If there was any resistance or concern that the tube is not positioned correctly, water-soluble contrast can be injected into the stomach via the new tube while taking an abdominal radiograph, which can confirm placement.[78]

SUMMARY

Postprocedural complications can occur after a wide variety of both inpatient and outpatient procedures. The severity of illness due to these complications is similarly wide, ranging from those that require simple supportive care to acutely life-threatening conditions. Although many postprocedural complications are closely temporally associated with their procedure, some may occur years later. A thorough history of surgical and procedural interventions is an important aspect of the evaluation of the emergency department patient, particularly those patients presenting with common symptoms of postprocedural complications including fever, abdominal pain, and wound complications.

CLINICS CARE POINTS

- Post-laparoscopic shoulder pain that persists beyond 72 hours or is accompanied by vital sign derangements is atypical and should prompt further evaluation.

- Unexplained tachycardia in an early post-bariatric surgery patient should raise concern for an anastomotic leak.
- Maturation of a gastrostomy tube tract occurs after approximately 1 month; blind reinsertion is contraindicated in immature tracts.

DISCLOSURE

The authors have nothing to disclose.

REFERENCES

1. Hall MJ, Schwartzman A, Zhang J, et al. Ambulatory Surgery Data From Hospitals and Ambulatory Surgery Centers: United States, 2010. Natl Health Stat Rep 2017; 102:1–15.
2. Paw P, Sackier JM. Complications of laparoscopy and thoracoscopy. J Intensive Care Med 1994;9(6):290–304.
3. Derouin M, Couture P, Boudreault D, et al. Detection of gas embolism by transesophageal echocardiography during laparoscopic cholecystectomy. Anesth Analg 1996;82(1):119–24.
4. Park EY, Kwon JY, Kim KJ. Carbon dioxide embolism during laparoscopic surgery. Yonsei Med J 2012;53(3):459–66.
5. Burcharth J, Burgdorf S, Lolle I, et al. Successful resuscitation after carbon dioxide embolism during laparoscopy. Surg Laparosc Endosc Percutan Tech 2012; 22(3):e164–7.
6. Kjeld T, Hansen EG, Holler NG, et al. Resuscitation by hyperbaric exposure from a venous gas emboli following laparoscopic surgery. Scand J Trauma Resusc Emerg Med 2012;20:1–5.
7. Taylor SP, Hoffman GM. Gas embolus and cardiac arrest during laparoscopic pyloromyotomy in an infant. Can J Anesth 2010;57(8):774–8.
8. Danwang C, Bigna JJ, Tochie JN, et al. Global incidence of surgical site infection after appendectomy: A systematic review and meta-analysis. BMJ Open 2020;10(2):1–7.
9. Sood S, Imsirovic A, Sains P, et al. Epigastric port retrieval of the gallbladder following laparoscopic cholecystectomy is associated with the reduced risk of port site infection and port site incisional hernia: An updated meta-analysis of randomized controlled trials: Gallbladder retrieval. Ann Med Surg 2020; 55(May):244–51.
10. Karthik S, Augustine AJ, Shibumon MM, et al. Analysis of laparoscopic port site complications: A descriptive study. J Minim Access Surg 2013;9(2):59–64.
11. Hamzaoglu I, Baca B, Böler DE, et al. Is umbilical flora responsible for wound infection after laparoscopic surgery? Surg Laparosc Endosc Percutan Tech 2004;14(5):263–7.
12. Fields AC, Lu P, Melnitchouk N. Reply: Does retrieval bag use during laparoscopic appendectomy reduce postoperative infection? Surg (United States) 2019;166(1):128.
13. Tanaka R, Kameyama H, Chida T, et al. Severe cellulitis and abdominal wall emphysema following laparoscopic colonic surgery: A case report. Asian J Endosc Surg 2015;8(2):193–6.
14. Valadan M, Banifatemi S, Yousefshahi F. Preoperative gabapentin to prevent postoperative shoulder pain after laparoscopic ovarian cystectomy: A randomized clinical trial. Anesthesiol Pain Med 2015;5(6):e31524.

15. Raval AD, Deshpande S, Koufopoulou M, et al. The impact of intra-abdominal pressure on perioperative outcomes in laparoscopic cholecystectomy: a systematic review and network meta-analysis of randomized controlled trials. Surg Endosc 2020;34(7):2878–90.

16. Sjövall S, Kokki M, Kokki H. Laparoscopic Surgery: A Narrative Review of Pharmacotherapy in Pain Management. Drugs 2015;75(16):1867–89.

17. Barrett M, Asbun HJ, Chien HL, et al. Bile duct injury and morbidity following cholecystectomy: a need for improvement. Surg Endosc 2018;32(4):1683–8.

18. Gouma DJ, Go PM. Bile duct injury during laparoscopic and conventional cholecystectomy. J Am Coll Surg 1994;178(3):229–33.

19. Bektas H, Schrem H, Winny M, et al. Surgical treatment and outcome of iatrogenic bile duct lesions after cholecystectomy and the impact of different clinical classification systems. Br J Surg 2007;94(9):1119–27.

20. Hindman NM, Arif-Tiwari H, Kamel IR, et al. ACR Appropriateness Criteria ® Jaundice. J Am Coll Radiol 2019;16(5):S126–40.

21. Fairchild AH, Hohenwalter EJ, Gipson MG, et al. ACR Appropriateness Criteria ® Radiologic Management of Biliary Obstruction. J Am Coll Radiol 2019;16(5): S196–213.

22. Solomkin JS, Mazuski JE, Bradley JS, et al. Diagnosis and management of complicated intra-abdominal infection in adults and children: Guidelines by the surgical infection society and the infectious diseases society of america. Clin Infect Dis 2010;50(2):133–64.

23. Masoomi H, Nguyen NT, Dolich MO, et al. Laparoscopic appendectomy trends and outcomes in the United States: Data from the Nationwide Inpatient Sample (NIS), 2004-2011. Am Surg 2014;80(10):1074–7.

24. Jaschinski T, Mosch CG, Eikermann M, et al. Laparoscopic versus open surgery for suspected appendicitis. Cochrane Database Syst Rev 2018;11(2):CD001546.

25. Gorter RR, Meiring S, van der Lee JH, et al. Intervention not always necessary in post-appendectomy abscesses in children; clinical experience in a tertiary surgical centre and an overview of the literature. Eur J Pediatr 2016;175(9):1185–91.

26. Scheirey CD, Fowler KJ, Therrien JA, et al. ACR Appropriateness Criteria ® Acute Nonlocalized Abdominal Pain. J Am Coll Radiol 2018;15(11):S217–31.

27. Kanona H, Al Samaraee A, Nice C, et al. Stump appendicitis: A review. Int J Surg 2012;10(9):425–8.

28. Hales CM, Carroll MD, Fryar CD, et al. Prevalence of Obesity Among Adults and Youth: United States, 2015–2016. NCHS data brief, no 288. Hyattsville, MD: National Center for Health Statistics. NCHS Data Brief 2017;(288):1–8.

29. English WJ, DeMaria EJ, Hutter MM, et al. American Society for Metabolic and Bariatric Surgery 2018 estimate of metabolic and bariatric procedures performed in the United States. Surg Obes Relat Dis 2020;16(4):457–63.

30. Colquitt JL, Pickett K, Loveman E, et al. Surgery for weight loss in adults. Cochrane Database Syst Rev 2014;2014(8).

31. Dayyeh BKA. Intragastric balloons for obesity management. Gastroenterol Hepatol 2017;13(12):737–9.

32. Kassir R, Debs T, Blanc P, et al. Complications of bariatric surgery: Presentation and emergency management. Int J Surg 2016;27:77–81.

33. Cho M, Pinto D, Carrodeguas L, et al. Frequency and management of internal hernias after laparoscopic antecolic antegastric Roux-en-Y gastric bypass without division of the small bowel mesentery or closure of mesenteric defects: review of 1400 consecutive cases. Surg Obes Relat Dis 2006;2(2):87–91.

34. Chand B, Prathanvanich P. Critical Care Management of Bariatric Surgery Complications. J Intensive Care Med 2016;31(8):511–28.

35. Luber SD, Fischer DR, Venkat A. Care of the Bariatric Surgery Patient in the Emergency Department. J Emerg Med 2008;34(1):13–20.

36. Carucci LR, Turner MA, Yu J. Imaging Evaluation Following Roux-en-Y Gastric Bypass Surgery for Morbid Obesity. Radiol Clin North Am 2007;45(2):247–60.

37. Mason EE, Hesson WW. Informed consent for obesity surgery. Obes Surg 1998; 8(4):419–28.

38. Moon RC, Teixeira AF, Goldbach M, et al. Management and treatment outcomes of marginal ulcers after Roux-en-Y gastric bypass at a single high volume bariatric center. Surg Obes Relat Dis 2014;10(2):229–34.

39. Lin YS, Chen MJ, Shih SC, et al. Management of Helicobacter pylori infection after gastric surgery. World J Gastroenterol 2014;20(18):5274–82.

40. Gumbs AA, Duffy AJ, Bell RL. Incidence and management of marginal ulceration after laparoscopic Roux-Y gastric bypass. Surg Obes Relat Dis 2006;2(4):460–3.

41. Wu Chao Ying V, Song SH, Khan K J, et al. Prophylactic PPI help reduce marginal ulcers after gastric bypass surgery: a systematic review and meta-analysis of cohort studies. Surg Endosc 2015;29(5):1018–23.

42. Dick A, Byrne TK, Baker M, et al. Gastrointestinal bleeding after gastric bypass surgery: Nuisance or catastrophe? Surg Obes Relat Dis 2010;6(6):643–7.

43. Braley SC, Nguyen NT, Wolfe BM. Late gastrointestinal hemorrhage after gastric bypass. Obes Surg 2002;12(3):404–7.

44. Saltzman E, Philip Karl J. Nutrient deficiencies after gastric bypass surgery. Annu Rev Nutr 2013;33:183–203.

45. Levy I, Gralnek IM. Complications of diagnostic colonoscopy, upper endoscopy, and enteroscopy. Best Pract Res Clin Gastroenterol 2016;30(5):705–18.

46. Reumkens A, Rondagh EJA, Bakker CM, et al. Post-colonoscopy complications: A systematic review, time trends, and meta-analysis of population-based studies. Am J Gastroenterol 2016;111(8):1092–101.

47. Quine MA, Bell GD, McCloy RF, et al. Prospective audit of perforation rates following upper gastrointestinal endoscopy in two regions of England. Br J Surg 1995;82(4):530–3.

48. Sieg A, Hachmoeller-Eisenbach U, Eisenbach T. Prospective evaluation of complications in outpatient GI endoscopy: A survey among German gastroenterologists. Gastrointest Endosc 2001;53(6):620–7.

49. Garbay JR, Suc B, Rotman N, et al. Multicentre study of surgical complications of colonoscopy. Br J Surg 1996;83(1):42–4.

50. Brinster CJ, Singhal S, Lee L, et al. Evolving options in the management of esophageal perforation. Ann Thorac Surg 2004;77(4):1475–83.

51. Kuppusamy MK, Hubka M, Felisky CD, et al. Evolving management strategies in esophageal perforation: Surgeons using nonoperative techniques to improve outcomes. J Am Coll Surg 2011;213(1):164–71.

52. Sawhney MS, Salfiti N, Nelson DB, et al. Risk factors for severe delayed postpolypectomy bleeding. Endoscopy 2008;40(2):115–9.

53. Pekgöz M. Post-endoscopic retrograde cholangiopancreatography pancreatitis: A systematic review for prevention and treatment. World J Gastroenterol 2019; 25(29):4019–42.

54. Kochar B, Akshintala VS, Afghani E, et al. Incidence, severity, and mortality of post-ERCP pancreatitis: A systematic review by using randomized, controlled trials. Gastrointest Endosc 2015;81(1):143–9.e9.

55. Adbel Aziz AM, Lehman GA. Pancreatits after endoscopic retrograde cholangio-pancreatography. World J Gastroenterol 2007;13(19):2655–68.
56. Dumonceau JM, Andriulli A, Elmunzer BJ, et al. Prophylaxis of post-ERCP pancreatitis: European society of gastrointestinal endoscopy (ESGE) guideline - Updated June 2014. Endoscopy 2014;46(9):799–815.
57. Gottlieb K, Sherman S, Pezzi J, et al. Early recognition of post-ERCP pancreatitis by clinical assessment and serum pancreatic enzymes. Am J Gastroenterol 1996; 91(8):1553–7.
58. Kaw M, Singh S. Serum lipase, c-reactive protein, and interleukin-6 levels in ERCP-induced pancreatitis. Gastrointest Endosc 2001;54(4):435–40.
59. Tenner S, Baillie J, Dewitt J, et al. American college of gastroenterology guideline: Management of acute pancreatitis. Am J Gastroenterol 2013;108(9):1400–15.
60. Sandø A, Rosen MJ, Heniford BT, et al. Long-term patient-reported outcomes and quality of the evidence in ventral hernia mesh repair: a systematic review. Hernia 2020;24(4):695–705.
61. Sharma R, Fadaee N, Zarrinkhoo E, et al. Why we remove mesh. Hernia 2018; 22(6):953–9.
62. Langbach O. Long term recurrence, pain and patient satisfaction after ventral hernia mesh repair. World J Gastrointest Surg 2015;7(12):384.
63. Kokotovic D, Bisgaard T, Helgstrand F. Long-term recurrence and complications associated with elective incisional hernia repair. JAMA 2016;316(15):1575–82.
64. Falagas ME, Kasiakou SK. Mesh-related infections after hernia repair surgery. Clin Microbiol Infect 2005;11(1):3–8.
65. Liang MK, Holihan JL, Itani K, et al. Ventral hernia management: Expert consensus guided by systematic review. Ann Surg 2017;265(1):80–9.
66. Niebuhr H, Köckerling F. Surgical risk factors for recurrence in inguinal hernia repair - A review of the literature. Innov Surg Sci 2020;2(2):53–9.
67. Petersen S, Henke G, Freitag M, et al. Deep prosthesis infection in incisional hernia repair: Predictive factors and clinical outcome. Eur J Surg 2001;167(6):453–7.
68. Taylor SG, O'Dwyer PJ. Chronic groin sepsis following tension-free inguinal hernioplasty. Br J Surg 1999;86(4):562–5.
69. Deysine M. Pathophysiology , Management of Prosthetic Infections in. Surg Clin North Am 1998;78(6):1105–15.
70. DeLegge MH. Enteral Access and Associated Complications. Gastroenterol Clin North Am 2018;47(1):23–37.
71. Hucl T, Spicak J. Complications of percutaneous endoscopic gastrostomy. Baillière's best practice & research. Clin Gastroenterol 2016;30(5):769–81. Available at: https://www.clinicalkey.es/playcontent/1-s2.0-S1521691816300804.
72. Lucendo AJ. Ana Belén Friginal-Ruiz. Percutaneous endoscopic gastrostomy: An update on its indications, management, complications, and care. Rev Esp Enferm Dig 2014;106(8):529–39.
73. Schrag SP, Sharma R, Jaik NP, et al. Complications related to percutaneous endoscopic gastrostomy (PEG) tubes. A comprehensive clinical review. J Gastrointest Liver Dis 2007;16(4):407–18. Available at: https://www.ncbi.nlm.nih.gov/pubmed/18193123.
74. El AZ, Arvanitakis M, Ballarin A, et al. Buried bumper syndrome: low incidence and safe endoscopic management. Acta Gastroenterol Bel 2011;74:312e6.
75. Cyrany J, Rejchrt S, Kopacova M, et al. Buried bumper syndrome: a complication of percutaneous endoscopic gastrostomy. World J Gastroenterol 2016;22: 618e27.

76. Chuang CH, Chen CY. Gastric herniation through PEG site. Gastrointest Endosc 2003;58:416.
77. Kaplan R, Delegge M. An unusual case of a ventral Richter's hernia at the site of a previous PEG tube. Dig Dis Sci 2006;51:2389e92.
78. Galat SA, Gerig KD, Porter JA, et al. Management of premature removal of the percutaneous gastrostomy. Am Surg 1990;56:733e6.

Occult Abdominal Trauma

Elizabeth Leenellett, MD[a],*, Adam Rieves, MD, MS[b]

KEYWORDS

- Blunt abdominal trauma • Occult injuries • Missed injuries

KEY POINTS

- Intraabdominal pathology from trauma can have a delayed presentation.
- Computed tomography is an imperfect imaging modality and can miss clinically relevant injuries.
- Patients that become unstable and have a suspicion for intraabdominal trauma should undergo diagnostic laparotomy.

DEFINING OCCULT ABDOMINAL TRAUMA

Several emergent medical conditions can be caused by occult abdominal trauma. In this article, we define an occult abdominal injury as an injury within the abdomen that is not diagnosed or suspected before a patient leaving the emergency department or an injury which is found in a patient that has a delayed presentation for care.

Maintaining a high index of suspicion for an occult injury can focus the history, physical examination, and workup to evaluate for these life-threatening conditions. For the purposes of this discussion, we exclude three major categories of injures. This discussion does not include hemodynamically unstable patients with blunt abdominal trauma and a positive Focused Assessment with Sonogram in Trauma (FAST) examination. These patients should undergo laparotomy.[1] Similarly, we will not discuss unstable patients with penetrating injuries to the abdomen as these patients also require laparotomy.[2] There are some conservative approaches to abdominal stab wounds that will be discussed toward the end of this article, however. Finally, this article will not address nontraumatic gastrointestinal bleeding.

Occult abdominal traumatic injuries can occur to any organ within the abdominal cavity. Patients with polytrauma are at risk for missed injuries because they may have other, more salient, life-threatening injuries. Other patients, however, can have delayed manifestations occurring hours to even days after a traumatic injury. Therefore, patients presenting to the emergency department with abdominal pain should be asked about even minor-seeming traumas to help elucidate the cause of their pain.

[a] Department of Emergency Medicine, University of Cincinnati, 231 Albert Sabin Way, Room 1505, Cincinnati, OH 45267-0769, USA; [b] Department of Emergency Medicine, Washington University in Saint Louis, 660 South Euclid Avenue, BC 8072, Saint Louis, MO 63110, USA
* Corresponding author.
E-mail address: leenele@ucmail.uc.edu

Emerg Med Clin N Am 39 (2021) 795–806
https://doi.org/10.1016/j.emc.2021.07.009
0733-8627/21/© 2021 Elsevier Inc. All rights reserved.

emed.theclinics.com

STATISTICS

According to the National Trauma Database (NTDB), abdominal trauma occurs in 11.7% of all injuries, mostly due to a blunt mechanism, and carries a 3.85% mortality rate.[3] Because not all hospitals report to the NTDB, these numbers likely underestimate the true prevalence of traumatic abdominal injuries. By its very definition, discerning the rate of occult abdominal trauma is difficult, especially when patients are initially evaluated, found to be without any abdominal pain or tenderness, discharged home, and later return with findings that result in hospitalization and potential surgical intervention. In a prospective observational study of patients with a worrisome blunt traumatic mechanism without any symptoms or signs of abdominal injury who underwent pan CT scans, clinically significant abnormalities were found on 7% of abdominal CT scans. Of those patients, 15% underwent laparotomy for hollow viscous and splenic injuries and 83% were admitted for serial examinations.[4] A recent retrospective analysis of asymptomatic trauma patients with concerning mechanisms of injury who underwent abdominal and pelvic CT revealed that 14% had positive CT scans and 1.1% underwent splenectomy.[5] This underscores the need for vigilance in screening for intraabdominal pathology and for a low threshold for diagnostic imaging because delays in diagnosis may lead to morbidity and mortality.[6–9]

RISK FACTORS

There are several factors that place patients at higher risk of an occult abdominal injury. Any condition that impairs the patient's ability to provide a complete and accurate history or impedes the clinician's ability to obtain a reliable physical examination enhances this risk. Examples of these conditions include altered mental status due to a variety of causes including concomitant head trauma or toxidrome, concomitant decompensated mental illness, dementia, and substance use. Additionally, pediatric patients may not be developmentally able to provide a history. Because nonaccidental trauma (NAT) is common and abused patients may have multiple injuries, screening for occult abdominal trauma should be part of any patient undergoing evaluation for NAT.[10]

Additional historical factors that may affect the risk of a missed intraabdominal injury (IAI) include medications like anticoagulants or antiplatelet agents, concurrent severe medical comorbidity, or recent illness. For example, a patient that is coagulopathic due to underlying disease or medication use is at risk for worse injury than a patient with normal clotting mechanisms and the same injury pattern. Special attention should be paid to patients who have recently had mononucleosis because splenic rupture has been reported up to 8 weeks from the onset of symptoms.[11]

COMMON MECHANISMS

Common blunt trauma mechanisms that are associated with occult IAI include motor vehicle collision (MVC), falls from a height, pedestrian struck by a vehicle, motorcycle collisions,[4] and bicycle accidents.[12,13] In general, falls and MVCs account for most deaths due to blunt trauma.[3] A meta-analysis of the literature from 2012 showed no relationship between the mechanism of blunt trauma (fall, MVC, and so forth) and the likelihood of IAI, although it was not specific to occult injuries.[14] According to a study by Parreira and colleagues,[15] pedestrians struck and motorcycle accidents account for the highest rate of occult abdominal trauma.

A direct blow from a steering wheel, the handlebars of a bicycle or motorcycle, or other object can cause compression and crush injuries to the solid and hollow organs, which can result in hemorrhage, viscus rupture, and peritonitis. Rapid deceleration injuries from substantial falls or MVCs can cause injury related to the movement of mobile organs that are tethered by their supporting ligaments. Examples include liver and spleen lacerations or hematomas and bucket handle injuries of the small bowel. Retroperitoneal injuries are also common in blunt abdominal trauma, are difficult to diagnose by physical examination, and can be missed by ultrasound.[16,17]

COMMONLY MISSED INJURIES

Essentially, any organ in the abdomen is at risk of an occult injury. Some injuries take time to declare themselves, such as posttraumatic pancreatitis, whereas other injuries may be missed because the mechanism required to cause them is associated with other, more salient, life-threatening injuries. Therefore, careful attention is required of patients who were initially well appearing after a seemingly minor trauma as well as to those who are severely injured with polytrauma to minimize the chance of missing a clinically significant IAI.

Blunt traumatic injuries can lacerate and potentially rupture the liver and spleen. As previously mentioned, infection with mononucleosis could heighten this risk as the spleen enlarges and lymphocytic infiltration threatens the structural integrity of the pulp and stretches the splenic capsule.[18] Cases of spontaneous splenic rupture in mononucleosis have been reported, but upon further questioning, an antecedent minor trauma is usually identified.[11]

Diaphragmatic injuries can occur due to either penetrating thoracoabdominal trauma or blunt abdominal trauma. These may be occult on CT. In a registry study of patients with occult abdominal injuries, 4% of the patients had a missed diaphragmatic injury.[19] Some diaphragmatic injuries may only be found on laparoscopy.

Hollow viscus injuries can occur and are difficult to diagnose. Although nearly any segment of the GI tract can be injured, ileal injuries are most common. These are highly morbid injuries because they allow contaminated GI contents to seed the peritoneal cavity and cause peritonitis.[20] Pancreatic and duodenal injuries can be difficult to diagnose and may have a delayed presentation. A handlebar injury is the classic mechanism for a duodenal injury.

Posttraumatic pancreatitis is possible, and it may take hours to days before the inflammation manifests following the injury.[21]

In anticoagulated patients especially, a minor traumatic event may lead to a retroperitoneal hematoma.[22]

Unexplained vital sign changes or an abdominal examination that does not fit with the patient's history or physical examination should prompt the clinician to consider evaluating the abdomen as a source of occult injury.

PHYSICAL EXAMINATION

Clinicians rely on the physical examination to determine which patients with trauma require imaging or prolonged observation. However, as previously discussed, those with altered mental status or those with concomitant distracting injuries can make the abdominal examination unreliable.[23-25] Furthermore, patients with isolated blunt abdominal trauma may present without complaints of abdominal pain or findings of abdominal tenderness despite having an IAI, which makes diagnosis extremely difficult.[5,24,26,27] As a result, multiple studies and clinical prediction rules have been proposed to ascertain which patients benefit from imaging. Nishijima and colleagues[14] conducted a meta-analysis of the literature in 2012 and found that IAI is more likely with examination findings of rebound tenderness (likelihood ratio range, 6.5; 95%

CI, 2.5%–8.6%), abdominal distention (LR, 3.8; 95% CI, 1.9–7.6), or guarding (LR, 3.7; 95% CI, 2.3–5.9). The authors also establish that the findings of a seat belt sign (LR, 5.6–9.9) and hypotension (LR, 5.2; 95% CI, 3.5–7.5) correlated with a higher likelihood of IAI which could potentially be seen in patients who present without complaints of abdominal pain. The presence of a femur fracture (LR, 2.9; 95% CI, 2.1–4.1) or costal margin tenderness after blunt thoracic injury also increases the likelihood of IAI given the forces required to break the ribcage, femur, or hip.[28,29] (**Box 1**).

LABORATORY FINDINGS

Several laboratories can be obtained to help identify an occult abdominal injury (**Box 2**).

- Unexplained anemia, especially in the setting of a delayed presentation, can suggest that a patient has a solid organ injury with ongoing bleeding.
- In one prospective study, a base deficit of more than −6 provided a probability of more than 95% for the absence of intraabdominal bleeding.[30]
- An elevated amylase or lipase level can occur concomitantly with a pancreatic injury and has been associated with hollow viscus injuries.
- Increased transaminases can help identify liver injury. Specifically, in pediatric patients, liver function tests in conjunction with abdominal examination can be used to justify a restrictive imaging strategy with cutoffs of AST greater than 200 IU/L or ALT greater than 125 IU/L.[31]
- Hematuria (>25 RBC/hpf) can help evaluate for a genitourinary injury and is associated with an increased risk for other IAIs.[28]

An abnormality in the laboratories described earlier should raise a provider's suspicion for an occult injury but in and of themselves do not require further workup. The decision to pursue advanced imaging or serial examinations should be based on a combination of factors including laboratories, history, physical examination, and any imaging that is already available.

IMAGING
Ultrasound

The FAST examination is recommended as the initial modality of choice for hemodynamically unstable patients with blunt abdominal trauma.[23] Multiple studies have been performed evaluating the sensitivity and specificity of ultrasound in detecting IAI.[1,32–34] It is rapid, inexpensive, and allows the patient to remain in the trauma bay to undergo continued resuscitation and evaluation simultaneously. However, it is

---

Box 1
Physical examination findings associated with intraabdominal injury

- Seat belt sign
- Rebound tenderness
- Hypotension
- Abdominal distention or guarding
- Hip or femur fracture
- Costal margin tenderness

Box 2
Laboratory values suggestive of occult abdominal injury

- Unexplained anemia
- Base deficit more than −6
- Elevated amylase or lipase
- ALT greater than 125 IU/L or AST greater than 200 IU/L
- Hematuria (>25 RBC/hpf)

---

dependent on provider experience, equipment, and the patient's body habitus and does not identify all injuries or the source of free intraabdominal fluid. Furthermore, a minimum fluid volume is required in order to be detected, which may take time to accumulate, and thus may not be visible on initial evaluation. Based on previous quantitative studies, most practitioners are unable to visualize free intraperitoneal fluid in the right upper quadrant until 600 cc has accumulated, although experienced clinicians may appreciate volumes as low as 400 cc.[35] Lobo and colleagues[36] found that the most sensitive area for visualizing free fluid on the FAST examination is the caudal tip of the liver. Free fluid in the pelvis can be visualized at much lower volumes with a median quantity of 100 cc.[37] Per Nishijima and colleagues,[14] a bedside ultrasound is more accurate in detecting fluid or organ injury than physical examination alone. For those patients without abdominal pain or tenderness but with a worrisome mechanism of injury, the FAST examination is a reasonable imaging option as a part of the evaluation for IAI.

Computerized Tomography

CT is a sensitive and specific diagnostic modality in detecting solid organ injuries in blunt abdominal trauma. It is rapid and provides information that may not be gleaned by ultrasound alone, including retroperitoneal, vascular, bony, and soft tissue evaluation. However, it does require transportation of the patient, is expensive, and has inherent risks of ionizing radiation, contrast nephropathy, contrast reactions, and may still miss subtle bowel, mesenteric, or diaphragmatic injuries. In addition, a reliable means of disclosing incidental findings such as pulmonary nodules or renal masses to the patient must be established.

For stable patients in whom occult IAI is a concern, the risks and benefits must be weighed. Clinical prediction rules to determine the utility of CT in patients with isolated blunt abdominal trauma have been studied.[15,24,28,29,38] Based on the consensus statement by ACEP, patients who do not have abdominal tenderness, altered mental status (GCS <14), costal margin tenderness, abnormal chest radiograph (CXR), hematocrit less than 30%, hematuria >/ = 25 RBCs/high power field, or hypotension are at low risk for IAI and may not need abdominal CT scanning (**Box 3**).[23] Rib fractures or pneumothorax found on CXR and hip or femur fractures are concerning for high impact injuries, may distract from a dependable abdominal examination, and have a higher correlation for IAI.[28,29,39]

Diagnostic Peritoneal Lavage

Diagnostic peritoneal lavage has been used in unstable patients with blunt abdominal trauma. It is sensitive in detecting intraperitoneal blood and bowel injury but is invasive and has risk for procedural complications. It is not used for detecting occult abdominal injury in hemodynamically stable patients.

Box 3
Criteria for selective CT imaging in blunt abdominal trauma

CT imaging may not be required if all of the following criteria are met for patients with isolated blunt abdominal trauma[23,28]:
- No abdominal tenderness
- Normal mental status
- No costal margin tenderness
- Normal CXR
- Hematocrit greater than 30%
- No hematuria
- No hypotension

MRI

MRI is a very sensitive and specific imaging modality for evaluating intraabdominal anatomy. However, given limited access in the emergency department, lengthy imaging times, difficulty with patient monitoring, and expense, it has limited usage in the emergency setting.

RATIONAL APPROACHES TO MINIMIZE RADIATION EXPOSURE

Whole-body imaging has been advocated to minimize risk of missed injuries.[4,40] However, given the concern for radiation exposure and long-term malignancy risk, an algorithm to minimize CT utilization would be beneficial. A review of the literature in 2013 found a paucity of randomized controlled trials that compared routine versus selective abdominal CT imaging in blunt trauma, and thus, a comparison of the morbidity and mortality of the two approaches was unable to be assessed.[41]

The findings from a retrospective review of patients with blunt abdominal trauma suggest that a rational approach for asymptomatic patients is observation with repeat evaluation of the patient over a period of time.[42] Specifically, they found that patients with significant IAI developed signs or symptoms within 9 hours of presentation. In fact, all patients requiring intervention developed signs or symptoms of IAI within 1 hour of arrival.[42] Freshman and colleagues[43] found that observation resulted in fewer overall numbers of CT scans and was cost effective. Two randomized controlled trials evaluating patients with a low index of suspicion for IAI found that a negative FAST examination was sufficient, decreasing the rate of abdominal CT utilization.[44,45]

Increased ED patient volumes, high acuity care, and boarding issues may also influence the decision to obtain advanced imaging studies. Although CT scans are time consuming to obtain and interpret, when balanced with resource management including physical space, personnel responsible for repeat abdominal examinations, fear of litigation for missed injuries, and the risk of developing abdominal pain or tenderness resulting in a delayed CT and a longer observation period, it may be more expedient to proceed directly to imaging, especially because studies show that patients with a negative CT can be discharged safely.[4,5,23,26,27,38,46,47] On the other hand, the clinical decision rules reviewed by ACEP provide a guideline for those who can avoid CT scanning altogether based on vital signs, physical examinations, CXR, and laboratory findings.[23] Each clinician must make that determination on a case-by-case basis based on experience, circumstance, resource availability, and comfort level.

DISPOSITION

Patients who have suspected or confirmed intraabdominal traumatic injuries have several possible dispositions from the emergency department. These can either be further diagnostic investigations, therapeutic interventions, observation, or discharge home.

As discussed in the introduction, patients who are hemodynamically unstable and have blunt or penetrating IAIs should go to the operating room for an exploratory laparotomy. In the operating theater, injuries can be clearly identified and intervened upon simultaneously. In an effort to decrease the morbidity associated with exploratory laparotomy, some centers have advocated for a laparoscopic approach to the evaluation of abdominal or thoracoabdominal trauma in certain cases.[48] This strategy can be particularly useful in identifying diaphragmatic tears. If the diagnostic question to be answered is only to evaluate for a diaphragmatic injury, such as a thoracoabdominal stab wound, laparoscopy alone can be a reasonable approach.[48,49]

The angiography suite can also serve as a useful destination for patients with IAIs. Specifically, patients with known solid organ injuries and evidence of ongoing bleeding can be managed with selective embolization compared with undergoing operative splenectomy or hepatorrhaphy.[50]

If a patient is not leaving the emergency department for emergent diagnostic or therapeutic intervention, the provider is left with the choice between discharge and observation. There is no single historical feature, physical examination finding, or laboratory finding that reliably rules out significant IAI. In a low-risk patient, a combination of clinical findings such as a normal physical examination in addition to normal laboratory results suggest a very low likelihood of IAI requiring no further evaluation.[14] Patients who have had a CT scan, and have normal vital signs, and a reassuring abdominal examination can be discharged with strict return precautions.

SPECIAL POPULATIONS
Pediatric Patients

Pediatric patients with abdominal trauma require special attention. Traumatic injuries are the most common cause of pediatric death, and blunt abdominal injuries are the most common unrecognized fatal injury.[51] Additionally, in pediatric patients, the solid organs are both relatively larger and less protected by the ribs than adult patients. This puts them at increased risk of injury from blunt trauma compared with adults.[52]

Controversy exists about an optimal diagnostic workup strategy for children with blunt abdominal trauma for several reasons. The FAST examination can help rule in an overt abdominal injury if free fluid is identified. However, half of all pediatric patients with an IAI will have a negative FAST examination.[53] Therefore, FAST examination alone cannot be used to rule out an IAI. Often, these patients will need to be observed with serial abdominal examinations to reassure providers that they do not have an occult abdominal injury. Imaging associated with ionizing radiation has better test characteristics for diagnosing IAI compared with ultrasonography, but the risks and benefits of this must be carefully weighed. As noted earlier, an algorithm incorporating liver function tests into the decision-making process can help optimize a pediatric patient's evaluation.

NAT is an unfortunately common mechanism of injury in pediatric patients. Consideration of NAT should be given to patients with acute abdominal symptoms; in patients with suspected NAT, a careful abdominal examination should be performed to risk stratify for additional injuries.[10] Patients with NAT often have multiorgan injuries, and in preverbal children, there may not be clues to raise one's index of suspicion for an IAI.

Pregnant Patients

Placental abruption can cause fetal demise and can be associated with even minor abdominal trauma. A particularly concerning aspect of placental abruption is its potential development up to 48 hours after an injury. The signs and symptoms can be subtle because patients can present with abdominal or pelvic pain and may or may not have associated vaginal bleeding. Ultrasound can be a useful tool to rule in abruption, but its sensitivity is not sufficient to rule out the diagnosis if it is not seen on ultrasound.[54] Therefore, these patients should be monitored with at least 6 hours of cardiotocographic monitoring.[55]

In pregnant patients, trauma is the leading cause of nonobstetric maternal mortality.[56] As with women who are not pregnant, CT is the test of choice for pregnant women in whom a severe injury is considered. If a CT scan is indicated to evaluate for an injury in a nonpregnant patient, then generally, the CT scan should be obtained in a pregnant patient; the actual decision for the provider is whether a CT scan is required in the first place. A fetal radiation dose of less than 50 mGy is not associated with increased fetal anomalies or fetal loss throughout pregnancy.[57] The estimated fetal radiation dose from conventional radiographic and CT examinations is well below this threshold. For example, a "pan scan" (CT head, c-spine, chest–abdomen–pelvis) exposes the fetus to an estimated total dose of 25.2 mGy—of which, 25 mGy is due to the abdomen/pelvis portion of the scan.[58] Therefore, the clinical decision-making around obtaining CT imaging in a pregnant patient should be framed in a similar way to a nonpregnant patient with the same injury pattern. The distance from the scanning beam to the fetus is the major driver of the fetal dose of radiation. A CT scan of the chest has less fetal radiation exposure than a plain film of the abdomen.[58]

These doses are cumulative, however, so careful consideration should be given to women who have already had evaluation with ionizing radiation in the same pregnancy (either repeated scans or repeated presentations for trauma). Time permitting, informed consent should be obtained before imaging.

SUMMARY

Providers should liberally screen for IAIs in any patient that may not be able to provide a complete and reliable history and examination. A worrisome mechanism of injury such as a motorcycle accident or pedestrian struck requires a higher level of vigilance, even if the patient denies abdominal pain or tenderness.

For those who have a benign examination but with a worrisome mechanism, the FAST examinations and/or observations are reasonable options when trying to avoid CT or admission. Review of the physical examination and laboratory findings associated with a higher correlation of IAI as well as the exclusion criteria for advanced imaging may aid in decision-making.

Children may benefit from a period of observation after a negative FAST examination when trying to avoid ionizing radiation. A careful abdominal examination is needed when there is suspicion for NAT.

If a female patient merits a CT scan based on clinical concern, then a CT should be obtained regardless of pregnancy status because fetal radiation doses are well below thresholds for increased risk of fetal anomaly or loss. Any patient with a viable pregnancy in the emergency department should be on cardiotocometry while in the emergency department to evaluate for signs of fetal distress.

CLINICS CARE POINTS

- When obtaining a history from a patient with abdominal pain, inquire about recent trauma.
- Patients with polytrauma should have a thorough investigation for concomitant occult abdominal injuries.
- CT imaging in a pregnant patient should not be avoided if it is the best modality to answer the clinical question at hand, similar to a nonpregnant patient.

DISCLOSURE

The authors have nothing to disclose.

REFERENCES

1. Stengel D, Rademacher G, Ekkernkamp A, et al. Emergency ultrasound-based algorithms for diagnosing blunt abdominal trauma. Cochrane Database Syst Rev 2015;(9):CD004446.
2. Como JJ, Bokhari F, Chiu WC, et al. Practice Management Guidelines for Selective Nonoperative Management of Penetrating Abdominal Trauma. J Trauma Acute Care Surg 2010;68(3):721–33.
3. American College of Surgeons, Committee on Trauma. National trauma Data bank report, 2016 2016. Available at: www.facs.org/-/media/files/quality-programs/trauma/ntdb/ntdb-annual-report-2016.ashx. Accessed January 20, 2021.
4. Salim A. Whole Body Imaging in Blunt Multisystem Trauma Patients Without Obvious Signs of Injury: Results of a Prospective Study. Arch Surg 2006; 141(5):468.
5. Neeki MM, Hendy D, Dong F, et al. Correlating abdominal pain and intra-abdominal injury in patients with blunt abdominal trauma. Trauma Surg Acute Care Open 2017;2(1):e000109.
6. Zingg T, Agri F, Bourgeat M, et al. Avoiding delayed diagnosis of significant blunt bowel and mesenteric injuries: Can a scoring tool make the difference? A 7-year retrospective cohort study. Injury 2018;49(1):33–41.
7. Fakhry SM, Brownstein M, Watts DD, et al. Relatively short diagnostic delays (<8 hours) produce morbidity and mortality in blunt small bowel injury: an analysis of time to operative intervention in 198 patients from a multicenter experience. J Trauma 2000;48(3):408–14 [discussion: 414–5].
8. Clarke JR, Trooskin SZ, Doshi PJ, et al. Time to Laparotomy for Intra-abdominal Bleeding from Trauma Does Affect Survival for Delays Up to 90 Minutes. J Trauma Inj Infect Crit Care 2002;52(3):420–5.
9. Malinoski DJ, Patel MS, Yakar DO, et al. A Diagnostic Delay of 5 Hours Increases the Risk of Death After Blunt Hollow Viscus Injury. J Trauma Inj Infect Crit Care 2010;69(1):84–7.
10. Lane WG, Dubowitz H, Langenberg P. Screening for occult abdominal trauma in children with suspected physical abuse. Pediatrics 2009;124(6):1595–602.
11. Bartlett A, Williams R, Hilton M. Splenic rupture in infectious mononucleosis: A systematic review of published case reports. Injury 2016;47(3):531–8.
12. Klin B, Efrati Y, Vaiman M, et al. Abdominal injuries following bicycle-related blunt abdominal trauma in children. Minerva Pediatr 2016;68(3):167–72.
13. Alkan M, Iskit SH, Soyupak S, et al. Severe Abdominal Trauma Involving Bicycle Handlebars in Children. Pediatr Emerg Care 2012;28(4):357–60.

14. Nishijima DK, Simel DL, Wisner DH, et al. Does this adult patient have a blunt intra-abdominal injury? JAMA 2012;307(14):1517–27.
15. Parreira JG, Malpaga JM, Olliari CB, et al. Predictors of "occult" intra-abdominal injuries in blunt trauma patients. Rev Col Bras Cir 2015;42(5):311–7.
16. American College of Surgeons. In: Advanced trauma life support: ATLS ; student course manual. 9th edition. American College of Surgeons; 2012.
17. Harris AC, Zwirewich CV, Lyburn ID, et al. Ct findings in blunt renal trauma. Radiographics 2001;21(Spec No):S201–14.
18. Smith EB, Custer RP. Rupture of the Spleen in Infectious Mononucleosis: A Clinicopathologic Report of Seven Cases. Blood 1946;1(4):317–33.
19. Parreira JG, Oliari CB, Malpaga JMD, et al. Severity and treatment of "occult" intra-abdominal injuries in blunt trauma victims. Injury 2016;47(1):89–93.
20. Tan K-K, Liu JZ, Go T-S, et al. Computed tomography has an important role in hollow viscus and mesenteric injuries after blunt abdominal trauma. Injury 2010; 41(5):475–8.
21. Debi U, Kaur R, Prasad KK, et al. Pancreatic trauma: A concise review. World J Gastroenterol 2013;19(47):9003–11.
22. Daliakopoulos SI, Bairaktaris A, Papadimitriou D, et al. Gigantic retroperitoneal hematoma as a complication of anticoagulation therapy with heparin in therapeutic doses: a case report. J Med Case Rep 2008;2:162.
23. Diercks DB, Mehrotra A, Nazarian DJ, et al. Clinical Policy: Critical Issues in the Evaluation of Adult Patients Presenting to the Emergency Department With Acute Blunt Abdominal Trauma. Ann Emerg Med 2011;57(4):387–404.
24. Richards JR, Derlet RW. Computed tomography for blunt abdominal trauma in the ED: a prospective study. Am J Emerg Med 1998;16(4):338–42.
25. Ferrera PC, Verdile VP, Bartfield JM, et al. Injuries distracting from intraabdominal injuries after blunt trauma. Am J Emerg Med 1998;16(2):145–9.
26. Benjamin E, Cho J, Recinos G, et al. Negative computed tomography can safely rule out clinically significant intra-abdominal injury in the asymptomatic patient after blunt trauma: Prospective evaluation of 1193 patients. J Trauma Acute Care Surg 2018;84(1):128–32.
27. Livingston DH, Lavery RF, Passannante MR, et al. Admission or Observation Is Not Necessary after a Negative Abdominal Computed Tomographic Scan in Patients with Suspected Blunt Abdominal Trauma: Results of a Prospective, Multi-institutional Trial. J Trauma Inj Infect Crit Care 1998;44(2):273–82.
28. Holmes JF, Wisner DH, McGahan JP, et al. Clinical prediction rules for identifying adults at very low risk for intra-abdominal injuries after blunt trauma. Ann Emerg Med 2009;54(4):575–84.
29. Shojaee M, Sabzghabaei A, Heidari A. Efficacy of new scoring system for diagnosis of abdominal injury after blunt abdominal trauma in patients referred to emergency department. Chin J Traumatol 2020;23(3):145–8.
30. Mofidi M, Hasani A, Kianmehr N. Determining the accuracy of base deficit in diagnosis of intra-abdominal injury in patients with blunt abdominal trauma. Am J Emerg Med 2010;28(8):933–6.
31. Holmes JF, Sokolove PE, Land C, et al. Identification of Intra-abdominal Injuries in Children Hospitalized Following Blunt Torso Trauma. Acad Emerg Med 1999;6(8): 799–806.
32. Hoff WS, Holevar M, Nagy KK, et al. Practice management guidelines for the evaluation of blunt abdominal trauma: the East practice management guidelines work group. J Trauma 2002;53(3):602–15.

33. McKenney MG, Martin L, Lentz K, et al. 1,000 Consecutive Ultrasounds for Blunt Abdominal Trauma. J Trauma Inj Infect Crit Care 1996;40(4):607–12.

34. Stengel D, Leisterer J, Ferrada P, et al. Point-of-care ultrasonography for diagnosing thoracoabdominal injuries in patients with blunt trauma. Cochrane Database Syst Rev 2018;(12):CD012669.

35. Branney SW, Wolfe RE, Moore EE, et al. Quantitative sensitivity of ultrasound in detecting free intraperitoneal fluid. J Trauma 1995;39(2):375–80.

36. Lobo V, Hunter-Behrend M, Cullnan E, et al. Caudal Edge of the Liver in the Right Upper Quadrant (RUQ) View Is the Most Sensitive Area for Free Fluid on the FAST Exam. West J Emerg Med 2017;18(2):270–80.

37. Von Kuenssberg Jehle D, Stiller G, Wagner D. Sensitivity in detecting free intraperitoneal fluid with the pelvic views of the FAST exam. Am J Emerg Med 2003; 21(6):476–8.

38. Poletti PA, Mirvis SE, Shanmuganathan K, et al. Blunt abdominal trauma patients: can organ injury be excluded without performing computed tomography? J Trauma 2004;57(5):1072–81.

39. Schurink GWH, Bode PJ, van Luijt PA, et al. The value of physical examination in the diagnosis of patients with blunt abdominal trauma: a retrospective study. Injury 1997;28(4):261–5.

40. Caputo ND, Stahmer C, Lim G, et al. Whole-body computed tomographic scanning leads to better survival as opposed to selective scanning in trauma patients: A systematic review and meta-analysis. J Trauma Acute Care Surg 2014;77(4): 534–9.

41. Van Vugt R, Keus F, Kool D, et al. Selective computed tomography (CT) versus routine thoracoabdominal CT for high-energy blunt-trauma patients. Cochrane Database Syst Rev 2013;(12):CD009743.

42. Jones EL, Stovall RT, Jones TS, et al. Intra-abdominal injury following blunt trauma becomes clinically apparent within 9 hours. J Trauma Acute Care Surg 2014; 76(4):1020–3.

43. Freshman SP, Wisner DH, Battistella FD, et al. Secondary survey following blunt trauma: a new role for abdominal CT scan. J Trauma 1993;34(3):337–40 [discussion: 340–1].

44. Rose JS, Levitt MA, Porter J, et al. Does the Presence of Ultrasound Really Affect Computed Tomographic Scan Use? A Prospective Randomized Trial of Ultrasound in Trauma. J Trauma Acute Care Surg 2001;51(3):545–50.

45. Melniker LA, Leibner E, McKenney MG, et al. Randomized controlled clinical trial of point-of-care, limited ultrasonography for trauma in the emergency department: the first sonography outcomes assessment program trial. Ann Emerg Med 2006;48(3):227–35.

46. Holmes JF, McGahan JP, Wisner DH. Rate of intra-abdominal injury after a normal abdominal computed tomographic scan in adults with blunt trauma. Am J Emerg Med 2012;30(4):574–9.

47. Barmparas G, Patel DC, Linaval NT, et al. A negative computed tomography may be sufficient to safely discharge patients with abdominal seatbelt sign from the emergency department: A case series analysis. J Trauma Acute Care Surg 2018;84(6):900–7.

48. D'Souza N, Bruce JL, Clarke DL, et al. Laparoscopy for occult left-sided diaphragm injury following penetrating thoracoabdominal trauma is both diagnostic and therapeutic. Surg Laparosc Endosc Percutaneous Tech 2016;26(1):e5–8.

49. Mahajna A, Mitkal S, Bahuth H, et al. Diagnostic laparoscopy for penetrating injuries in the thoracoabdominal region. Surg Endosc 2004;18(10):1485–7.

50. Stassen NA, Bhullar I, Cheng JD, et al. Nonoperative management of blunt hepatic injury: an Eastern Association for the Surgery of Trauma practice management guideline. J Trauma Acute Care Surg 2012;73(5 Suppl 4):S288–93.
51. Cantor RM, Leaming JM. Evaluation and Management of Pediatric Major Trauma. Emerg Med Clin North Am 1998;16(1):229–56.
52. Bachur RG, Shaw KN. Fleisher & Ludwig's textbook of pediatric emergency medicine. In: Bachur RG, Shaw KN, editors. 7th edition. Lippincott Williams & Wilkins; 2015.
53. Holmes JF, Gladman A, Chang CH. Performance of abdominal ultrasonography in pediatric blunt trauma patients: a meta-analysis. J Pediatr Surg 2007;42(9): 1588–94.
54. Shinde GR, Vaswani BP, Patange RP, et al. Diagnostic Performance of Ultrasonography for Detection of Abruption and Its Clinical Correlation and Maternal and Foetal Outcome. J Clin Diagn Res 2016;10(8):QC04–7.
55. Barraco RD, Chiu WC, Clancy TV, et al. Practice Management Guidelines for the Diagnosis and Management of Injury in the Pregnant Patient: The EAST Practice Management Guidelines Work Group. J Trauma Acute Care Surg 2010;69(1): 211–4.
56. Fildes J, Reed L, Jones N, et al. Trauma: the leading cause of maternal death. - Abstract - Europe PMC. J Trauma Inj Infect Crit Care 1992;32(5):643–5.
57. Guidelines for diagnostic imaging during pregnancy and lactation. Committee Opinion No. 723. American College of Obstetricians and Gynecologists. Obstet Gynecol 2017;130:e210–6.
58. Raptis CA, Mellnick VM, Raptis DA, et al. Imaging of Trauma in the Pregnant Patient. RadioGraphics 2014;34(3):748–63.

Abdominal Pain in the Immunocompromised Patient

Carmen Wolfe, MD[a],*, Nicole McCoin, MD[b]

KEYWORDS

- Abdominal pain • Immunocompromise • Transplant • Malignancy • HIV/AIDS

KEY POINTS

- A careful history should be taken to identify patients with congenital, acquired, and medication-induced immunodeficiencies.
- Classic physical examination findings of a serious pathologic abdominal condition may be absent in immunocompromised patients despite the presence of significant abnormalities.
- A differential diagnosis should be constructed by considering the patient's cause of immunocompromise, as well as the most likely emergencies associated with their underlying condition or medication.
- Laboratory testing should be broad, and cross-sectional imaging should be liberally used.
- A more conservative approach regarding disposition is prudent in this high-risk group.

INTRODUCTION

Abdominal pain carries a broad differential diagnosis, and in patients with compromised immune systems unusual conditions and opportunistic infections can be more common. Emergency department (ED) evaluation relies first on the recognition of immunocompromise in these individuals, whether due to congenital, acquired, or medication-induced causes, followed by careful consideration of a broader differential than typically entertained in an immunocompetent patient.

HISTORY

A careful history is essential in the identification of an immunocompromised state. Classic categories of immunocompromise include oncology patients undergoing

[a] Department of Emergency Medicine, Vanderbilt University Medical Center, 1313 21st Avenue South, Oxford House 703, Nashville, TN 37232, USA; [b] Department of Emergency Medicine, Ochsner Medical Center, 1514 Jefferson Highway, New Orleans, LA 70121, USA
* Corresponding author.
E-mail address: carmenwolfe@gmail.com

Emerg Med Clin N Am 39 (2021) 807–820
https://doi.org/10.1016/j.emc.2021.07.002
0733-8627/21/© 2021 Elsevier Inc. All rights reserved.
emed.theclinics.com

chemotherapy, posttransplant patients, and patients with human immunodeficiency virus (HIV)/acquired immunodeficiency syndrome (AIDS). However, beyond these broad categories, there are many other factors to consider when determining if a patient is immunocompromised. Particular attention to past medical history, family history, and medications is crucial to identify a larger breadth of immunocompromised patients including congenital immunodeficiency disorders, acquired immunodeficiencies, and the use of immunosuppressive medications.

A primary immunodeficiency may be suggested by a history of recurrent severe infections or by infections with unusual or opportunistic organisms. Congenital immunodeficiency disorders can affect B cells, T cells, neutrophils, phagocytes, complement, or a combination of immune cell lines.[1] Selective immunoglobulin IgA deficiency is the most common primary pediatric and adult immunodeficiency.[2] In the absence of an established diagnosis, primary immunodeficiency may be suggested by a family history of primary immunodeficiency, a history of recurrent severe infections, or by infections with unusual or opportunistic organisms.

Acquired immunodeficiency is classically associated with HIV infection and the development of AIDS. HIV targets CD4 T cells, which play a vital role in the regulation of the immune response, making individuals susceptible to a host of opportunistic infections. Pathogens associated with opportunistic infections are closely linked to the degree of immunosuppression, commonly estimated based on the CD4 count.[3] Knowledge of a patient's CD4 count can guide physicians in diagnosis and empirical management. The CD4 count may be directly reported by many hospital laboratories; however, due to lengthy turnaround times it is often unavailable at the time of the initial ED encounter or in resource-limited settings.[4] In these instances, the CD4 count may be estimated based on the patient's absolute lymphocyte count (ALC).[5] In one study, an ALC of less than 1000 cell/mm^3 predicted a CD4 count less than 200 cell/mm^3 with 67% sensitivity and 96% specificity, and it can serve as a lower threshold to suggest significant immunocompromise. To rule out significant immunocompromise, an ALC cutoff of less than 2000 cell/mm^3 may be used; this improves the sensitivity to 97%, whereas the specificity drops to 41%.[5] CD4 counts of less than 200 are associated with severe immunosuppression and increased risk of opportunistic infections, including those responsible for gastrointestinal (GI) disease.[3]

In addition to HIV/AIDS, other conditions associated with a degree of acquired immunodeficiency include diabetes, uremia, and malnutrition.[6] Hyperglycemia associated with diabetes mellitus is known to cause immune dysfunction and increased susceptibility to infection.[6,7] This mechanism is multifaceted and includes impairment of cytokine production, leukocyte recruitment inhibition, defects in pathogen recognition, neutrophil dysfunction, dysfunction of both phagocytosis and chemotaxis of macrophages, natural killer cell dysfunction, poor lymphoproliferative response, and abnormal compliment activation.[6,7] Patients with chronic kidney disease are functionally immunocompromised due to defective renal metabolic activities and impaired glomerular filtration resulting in the accumulation of uremic toxins. Dysfunction and altered apoptotic rates of polymorphonuclear leukocytes, monocytes, and lymphocytes lead to an impaired immune response and increased susceptibility to infection.[8] Malnutrition confers an inherent immunodeficiency due to impaired immune priming and memory T cell function, among other complex mechanisms. This impairment has demonstrated a clear link to increased mortality from infectious disease.[9] Concern for malnutrition may be raised by the patient or family members or may be suspected based on objective data from historical and current weight measurements. Elderly patients are at risk for malnutrition, particularly those with dysphagia, Parkinson's disease, cognitive decline, dementia, frailty, excessive polypharmacy, and institutionalization.[10] Additional populations at risk for malnutrition include patients with a history of alcohol use disorder, GI disease-associated malabsorption, developmental disorders, mental health disorders, cancer, and a history of previous bariatric surgery.

Medication-induced immunocompromise is associated with a broad array of medications prescribed to many diverse patient populations including oncology patients, posttransplant patients, and patients with autoimmune disease among others. Oncology patients may be taking traditional chemotherapeutic agents or novel monoclonal antibody immune checkpoint inhibitors. Although chemotherapeutic agents represent a heterogeneous group of medications, a large majority of these depress the patient's immune system, with or without the presence of neutropenia. Immune checkpoint inhibitors treat cancer by blocking binding of checkpoint proteins that typically downregulate the immune system, thereby allowing T cells to target and destroy cancer cells.[11] This group of medications causes an upregulation of the immune response, whereas it can paradoxically increase a patient's susceptibility to infection due to immunosuppressants given to treat immune-related adverse events that are common with these medications.[12] After organ transplantation, patients are treated with medication to specifically suppress their immune system and prevent rejection of the transplanted organ. The particular immunosuppressant regimen depends on the transplanted organ and varies widely across transplant programs. For kidney transplants, the most common regimen includes tacrolimus and prednisone with mycophenolic acid or azathioprine; other regimens include steroid-sparing, mycophenolic acid/azathioprine-sparing, mammalian target of rapamycin-based, and cyclosporine-based regimens.[13] Patients with autoimmune disease may be taking specific immunomodulators or high-dose steroids to suppress their underlying disease, affecting their expected immune response to any infection. Monoclonal antibodies are often used to suppress immune activity to treat common autoimmune disorders such as rheumatoid arthritis, multiple sclerosis, systemic lupus erythematosus, psoriasis, and inflammatory bowel disease. The mechanism of action of these monoclonal antibodies varies depending on the specific agent, but in general targets T cell and B cell lymphocyte surface proteins and leads to increased susceptibility to infection.[14]

Although oncology patients, posttransplant patients, and patients with autoimmune disease are the most commonly encountered groups of patients taking immunosuppressants, this category of medications is broad and is indicated in a variety of other conditions as well. Monoclonal antibodies have been used to treat patients with age-related macular degeneration,[15] hidradenitis suppurativa,[16] persistent allergic asthma,[17] chronic rhinosinusitis,[18] paroxysmal nocturnal hemoglobinuria,[19] and coronavirus disease 2019.[20] Thus, a specific review of the patient's medications should reveal key clues that might aid in diagnosis. Medication list review may also identify drugs attributing to a patient's presenting symptoms either due to potential side effects of the drug, including nausea, vomiting, or abdominal pain, or due to specific downstream diagnoses associated with the drug, including pancreatitis, gastritis, or gastric ulcers.

PHYSICAL EXAMINATION

As with all patients with abdominal pain, a thorough physical examination is crucial in the evaluation of the immunocompromised patient with abdominal pain. A common portion of the physical examination that is often neglected or purposefully excluded in neutropenic patients is the digital rectal examination (DRE). Consensus recommendations cosponsored by multiple organizations recommend against DREs, stating concern that DRE may cause skin or mucosal breakdown and promote bacterial translocation; however, this recommendation is a moderate strength recommendation based on poor-quality evidence (category DIII).[21] Anorectal disease is an important source of sepsis to consider in patients with malignancy and confers a high mortality when present. Identification of this pathologic condition is crucial in patients presenting with undifferentiated sepsis and should be considered.[21]

Immunocompromised patients may lack a robust immune response to underlying pathologic conditions thus decreasing the presence of associated inflammation and the expected physical examination findings. Although the presence of tenderness is helpful to raise one's suspicion of significant intra-abdominal pathologic condition, its absence should not indicate the opposite. The information gleaned in the physical examination should be used to augment a list of pathologic possibilities but should not be used to exclude them.

DIFFERENTIAL DIAGNOSIS

The differential diagnosis for abdominal pain in the immunocompromised patient is broad because it includes both diagnoses encountered throughout the healthy population and those specific to the immunocompromised population. In evaluation of an immunocompromised patient, consideration of the underlying cause of the immunocompromise can assist the ED clinician in formulating an appropriate differential diagnosis, choosing appropriate diagnostic testing, and providing appropriate treatments. Important conditions to consider include congenital immunodeficiencies, malignancy, hematopoietic stem cell transplant, solid organ transplant (SOT), and HIV/AIDS.

CONGENITAL IMMUNODEFICIENCIES

Congenital immunodeficiencies can lead to a wide variety of GI manifestations as gut-associated lymphoid tissue is the largest lymphoid organ in the body with multiple mechanisms for immune regulation. Each congenital immunodeficiency places the patient at risk for particular types of infections and GI complications depending on the pathogenesis of disease. The most common congenital immunodeficiencies and their associated complications that may lead to the presenting symptom of abdominal pain can be found in **Fig. 1**. Diarrhea and malabsorption are particularly common in this subset of patients.[22]

MALIGNANCY

Although mucositis, neutropenic enterocolitis, and structural causes (obstruction, intussusception, perforation) of abdominal pain can be seen in other immunocompromised states, they are particularly common in the setting of malignancy. These and other causes of abdominal pain in the patient with a diagnosis of malignancy are denoted in **Fig. 1**. Allogenic stem cell transplant recipients can develop graft-versus-host disease (GVHD), discussed in detail in the section focusing on hematopoietic stem cell transplantation.

Mucositis

Mucositis can extend far beyond the familiar oral mucositis to affect any area of the GI tract. The incidence of GI mucositis varies widely based on the chemotherapeutic regimen but can affect up to 80% of patients.[23] GI mucositis can present with abdominal pain and diarrhea. This condition is caused by chemotherapy, radiation, or a

Congenital Immunodeficiencies	Malignancy	Hematopoietic Stem Cell Transplantation	Solid Organ Transplantation	HIV/AIDS
IgA Deficiency	Bacterial Infection (Clostridium difficile; Campylobacter; Salmonella; Shigella; E coli; Yersinia; Vibrio)	Bacterial Infection (Clostridium difficile; Campylobacter; Salmonella; Shigella; E coli; Yersinia; Vibrio)	Bacterial Infection (Clostridium difficile; Campylobacter; Salmonella; Shigella; E coli; Yersinia; Vibrio)	Bacterial Infection (Clostridium difficile; Campylobacter; Salmonella; Shigella; MAI)
Giardia Lamblia Infection	Viral Infection (CMV; HSV; VZV; Adenovirus; Norwalk)	Viral Infection (CMV; HSV; VZV; Adenovirus; Norwalk)	Viral Infection (CMV; HSV; VZV; Adenovirus; Norwalk)	Viral Infection (coinfection with Hepatitis B and C; CMV; HSV; Adenovirus; Rotavirus; Norovirus)
Celiac Disease	Fungal Infection (Histoplasmosis; Coccidiomycosis; Cryptococcus; Candidiasis)	Fungal Infection (Histoplasmosis; Coccidiomycosis; Cryptococcus; Candidiasis)	Fungal Infection (Histoplasmosis; Coccidiomycosis; Cryptococcus; Candidiasis)	Fungal Infection (Histoplasmosis; Coccidiomycosis; Cryptococcus; Candidiasis)
Chronic Hepatitis	Parasitic Infection (Cryptosporidium; Cyclospora; Entamoeba histolytica)	Parasitic Infection (Cryptosporidium; Cyclospora; Entamoeba histolytica)	Parasitic Infection (Cryptosporidium; Cyclospora; Entamoeba histolytica)	Parasitic Infection (Cryptosporidium; Microsporidia; Giardia lamblia; Entamoeba histolytica)
Inflammatory Bowel Disease	Mucositis	Mucositis	Malignancy (Kaposi Sarcoma; Post-transplantation Lymphoproliferative Disorder)	Malignancy (Kaposi's Sarcoma, Non-Hodgkin's lymphoma, Leiomyoma, Rhabdomyosarcoma, High-Grade Pleomorphic Sarcoma, and GI Stromal Tumor)
Common Variable Immunodeficiency	Necrotizing Enterocolitis	Graft Versus Host Disease	Mucosal ulceration	Gastrointestinal Bleed
Salmonella Infection	Gastrointestinal Bleeding	Gastrointestinal Bleed	Graft Versus Host Disease	Intestinal Obstruction
Campylobacter Infection	Intussusception	Intestinal Obstruction	Gastrointestinal Bleed	Perforation
Norovirus Infection	Obstruction	Perforation	Intestinal Obstruction	Biliary Tract Disease (Sclerosing Cholangitis associated with Opportunistic Infections or Acalculous Cholecystitis associated with CMV)
Cytomegalovirus Infection	Perforation	Biliary Tract Disease	Perforation (especially Lung Transplant)	Pancreatitis
Giardia Lamblia Infection	Biliary Tract Disease	Pancreatitis	Biliary Tract Disease	Appendicitis (Associated with CMV)
Malignancy (especially Gastric Cancer; Lymphoma)	Pancreatitis	Diverticular Disease	Pancreatitis	HAART Adverse Effects
Hepatitis	Diverticular Disease	Appendicitis	Diverticular Disease (especially Renal Transplant)	AIDS Enteropathy
Biliary Disease	Appendicitis	Ischemic Colitis	Appendicitis	
Granulomatous Disease of the GI Tract	Ischemic Colitis	Chemotherapy/Radiation Related Complications	Ischemic Colitis (especially Renal Transplant)	
Inflammatory Bowel Disease			Immunosuppressive Drug Related Complications	
Severe Combined Immunodeficiency			Post-Operative Complications Related to Specific Type of Transplant	
Salmonella Infection				
E coli Infection				
Cryptosporidium Infection				
Adenovirus Infection				
Picornavirus Infection				
Parvovirus Infection				
Giardia Lamblia Infection				

Fig. 1. Causes of Abdominal Pain in Various Immunocompromised States. CMV, cytomegalovirus; HAART, highly active antiretroviral therapy; HSV, herpes simplex virus; MAI, mycobacterium avium-intracellulare; VZV, varicella zoster virus.

combination of both. Patients with mucositis in the small intestine and colon have multiple findings including crypt hypoplasia, altered goblet cell distribution, changes in mucin composition, and altered absorptive function.[24] GI bleeding is significantly more common during chemotherapy cycles associated with GI mucositis versus chemotherapy cycles without GI mucositis (13% vs 8%; $P = .04$).[25] Mucositis additionally increases the risk of infection of abdominal origin, sepsis, and septic shock.[26] Infection is significantly more common during chemotherapy cycles associated with GI mucositis versus chemotherapy cycles without GI mucositis (73% vs 36%; $P<.0001$).[25]

Neutropenic Enterocolitis

Neutropenic enterocolitis is known by several names: typhlitis, neutropenic colitis, necrotizing enterocolitis, ileocecal syndrome, and cecitis. Neutropenic enterocolitis can be seen in patients with acute myelogenous leukemia or acute lymphocytic leukemia before chemotherapy, in patients on chemotherapy, and in patients with other causes of immunosuppression, such as AIDS or posttransplantation. However, it is most commonly discussed when forming a differential diagnosis for the neutropenic patient with cancer because it is the most common cause of the acute abdomen in that population.[27] Although the pathogenesis of this disease is likely multifactorial, it is established that cytotoxicity of chemotherapy to the bowel mucosa and microbial invasion of the injured mucosa play a major role.[27] Initially, this disease process was thought to only involve the ileocecal region due to its poor vascularity and increased distension; however, involvement throughout other areas of the colon occurs in as many as 75% cases.[28] The onset of symptoms is typically 3 weeks into chemotherapy treatment correlating to the onset of mucosal damage. Patients present with the triad of neutropenia (absolute neutrophil count $<500 \times 10^9$ cells/L), fever, and abdominal pain. Diarrhea and lower GI bleeding can also be present. Although this diagnosis may be suspected based on these presenting signs and symptoms, computed tomography of the abdomen with intravenous contrast is typically used to confirm this diagnosis and may reveal thickening of the bowel wall, dilation of the colon, pericolonic inflammation, or pneumatosis intestinalis.[29] Ultrasonography may also be considered to aid in diagnosis, particularly in pediatric patients, with a sonographic measurement of bowel wall thickness of greater than 10 mm correlating to a higher mortality rate.[30] Clostridium difficile infection and GVHD (in those with hematopoietic stem cell transplant) should be ruled out as well. Complications of neutropenic enterocolitis include bacteremia, hemorrhage, and bowel wall perforation. Surgical intervention may be necessary.[28]

Structural Pathologies

Obstructions of both the small and large bowel are observed more frequently in patients with cancer. For example, the frequency of obstruction in patients with colorectal cancer is 10% to 28% per year and is 20% to 50% per year in those with ovarian cancer. Breast cancer and melanoma are the most common non-intra-abdominal cancers to cause bowel obstruction, usually due to peritoneal carcinomatosis.[31] The obstruction can occur due to intraluminal growth of tumor, intramural infiltration of tumor, or extramural compression of tumor, affected nodes, or adhesions. Tumor can also infiltrate into the mesentery and affect bowel wall muscles and nerves leading to functional obstruction. Functional obstruction can also be caused by pain medications or paraneoplastic neuropathy, particularly in patients with lung cancer.

Intussusception is less common in adults. However, when it does occur in the adult population, solid tumors are the lead point in more than 65% of intussusception cases.[32] Bowel perforation can result from a variety of the diagnoses discussed earlier including bowel obstructions, neutropenic enterocolitis, and progression of infection, as well as erosion of the bowel wall by either primary GI tumors or metastatic lesions to the GI tract.

HEMATOPOIETIC STEM CELL TRANSPLANT

Hematopoietic stem cell transplants are a treatment option for patients with a variety of disease processes including hematologic malignancies, such as lymphoma and leukemia, bone marrow failure syndromes, various immune deficiencies, as well as emerging use in the treatment of sickle cell disease.[33] In preparation for the stem cell transplant, a conditioning regimen that may include high-dose chemotherapy, monoclonal antibody therapy, and radiation is administered. The conditioning regimen itself, particularly highly cytotoxic chemotherapeutic regimens, can cause a host of problems as noted earlier. However, two important complications observed in patients with hematopoietic stem cell transplantation are acute GVHD and cytomegalovirus (CMV) infection. GVHD, CMV infection, and other causes of abdominal pain in the patient who is a recipient of a hematopoietic stem cell transplant are listed in **Fig. 1**.

Graft-Versus-Host Disease

GVHD is a condition in which immune cells from the donor attack healthy recipient tissues. The GI system is one of the most common sites of GVHD, and it can affect any segment of the GI tract. Early symptoms include anorexia, early satiety, and dyspepsia, progressing to nausea, vomiting, abdominal pain, diarrhea that can be quite profound, and GI bleeding. As these symptoms are nonspecific, consideration of the timing of symptom onset in reference to conditioning therapy and engraftment can help narrow the differential. Engraftment typically occurs at approximately 2 weeks. Therefore, symptoms occurring within this time frame are more suggestive of acute GVHD,[34] whereas symptoms occurring before engraftment of foreign stem cells are more likely attributable to chemotherapy-induced toxicity and opportunistic infections. In addition, radiographic appearance and location of the affected portion of the GI tract may aid in diagnosis. Minimal wall thickening less than 5 mm with significant mucosal enhancement is more commonly seen in computed tomographic imaging of patients with GVHD, in contrast to the thicker bowel wall seen in neutropenic enterocolitis. In addition, small intestinal involvement is present in approximately 75% of cases of GVHD, which aids in the exclusion of pathologic condition such as *C difficile* colitis. However, these are simply aids in narrowing the differential and are not definitive.[28] It is not uncommon for drug toxicity, infections, and acute GVHD to coexist.[34] Further investigation to differentiate the cause of the abdominal pain beyond the initial workup in the ED is necessary.

Cytomegalovirus Infection

There is reliable risk of CMV reactivation in patients with solid cancer[35]; however, it is of particular concern in patients with hematologic malignancies and hematopoietic stem cell transplantation. CMV causes multiorgan disease. GI CMV disease, typically presenting with fever, abdominal pain, and diarrhea that is often bloody, is the most frequently diagnosed type involving 70% to 80% of all cases.[36] This disease leads to mucosal ulcers throughout the GI tract, often with secondary bleeding and potential perforation. CMV polymerase chain reaction (PCR) testing has limited utility in the diagnosis of CMV colitis because half of the patients with GI CMV disease may have a negative serum PCR result early in the course of illness.[37] Endoscopy or colonoscopy with biopsy provides a more definitive diagnosis for GI CMV disease.[38] Histologic findings can also mimic acute GVHD, so immunohistochemical staining and viral culture of biopsied tissue are often performed.[34]

SOLID ORGAN TRANSPLANTATION

GI complications occur in approximately 40% of patients who are recipients of SOT.[36] Many of these complications overlap with those seen in other immunocompromised states, such as infections (particularly CMV and herpesvirus) and GVHD (less commonly with SOT than with hematopoietic stem cell transplant). Immunosuppressant medications and posttransplantation lymphoproliferative disorder (PTLD) are 2 potential causes of GI emergencies that are more unique to this subset of patients. **Fig. 1** lists these and other causes of abdominal pain in the patient with a SOT.

Immunosuppressant Medications

Tacrolimus, cyclosporine, sirolimus, mycophenolate mofetil, azathioprine, and steroids are some of the most common immunosuppressant medications prescribed after SOT. Although immunosuppressant therapies significantly decrease the rates of transplant rejection, they are associated with significant side effects and account for more than 50% of transplant-related deaths.[39]

Azathioprine use is associated with increased risk of hepatotoxicity.[40] Cyclosporine use has been associated with the formation of gallstones.[41] Azathioprine, cyclosporine, tacrolimus, and steroids have been associated with the development of pancreatitis.[40]

Steroid administration is associated with risk of GI bleeding or perforation. In addition, the clinician must use a cautious approach when evaluating patients taking steroids because this class of medications frequently masks symptoms of other GI disorders and can delay diagnosis and treatment.

Two-thirds of patients with SOT experience medication-associated diarrhea, most often with tacrolimus, sirolimus, and mycophenolate mofetil. Noninfectious diarrhea has been associated with increased risk of graft loss and mortality. Nausea, vomiting, and anorexia may also occur with the use of these medications.

Generalized abdominal pain has been associated with tacrolimus, sirolimus, and mycophenolate mofetil. In fact, up to 19% of patients who receive mycophenolate mofetil report abdominal pain. Drug-related abdominal pain would be a diagnosis of exclusion in the workup of these patients, but it does indeed exist.[40]

Posttransplant Lymphoproliferative Disorder

SOT increases risk of malignancy. Certain malignancies that are uncommon in the general population are more common in patients with SOT. Some examples include skin cancers, Kaposi sarcoma, and PTLDs.[41] PTLD ranges from benign hyperplasia to lymphoma and can occur in up to 10% of all SOT recipients. Incidence varies widely depending on the type of organ transplant and age of the patient, with higher rates seen in pediatric populations than in adults. Higher rates are seen in small bowel, heart, and lung transplant when compared with liver or kidney transplant.[42] Incidence is highest in the first year after transplant and declines thereafter.[43] The term PTLD refers to a clinically and pathologically diverse group of tumors, although it is most commonly linked to Epstein-Barr virus (EBV)-associated B lymphocyte proliferation.[44] Patients can present with fever, malaise, and respiratory symptoms. If PTLD affects the GI tract, obstruction, bleeding, or perforation may be seen.[36] Even though there is a strong relationship between EBV-induced B cell proliferation and PTLD, some patients who develop this disorder test negative for the virus. The diagnosis of PTLD may be suspected clinically based on symptoms and time of onset after transplant, but definitive diagnosis requires biopsy. Mortality for PTLD is high, often exceeding 50%, and represents the most common cause of cancer-related death after SOT.[43]

HUMAN IMMUNODEFICIENCY VIRUS/ACQUIRED IMMUNE DEFICIENCY SYNDROME
Infectious Causes

Abdominal pain may be caused by AIDS-related sclerosing cholangitis, which can be caused by several different opportunistic infections including microsporidia, cryptosporidia, and CMV. CMV infection, as previously discussed, may cause colitis or may be associated with acalculous cholecystitis or appendicitis as well.

Abdominal pain with diarrhea in the patient with HIV/AIDS may be caused by pathogens that can also be seen in immunocompetent patients. Nontyphoidal *Salmonella*, *Shigella*, *Yersinia*, and *Campylobacter* can occur with fever, nausea, abdominal pain, and bloody diarrhea. *C difficile* infection is more than 2-fold more common in HIV-positive patients. In fact, it is the most common infectious cause of diarrhea in hospitalized HIV-positive patients.[45] Viral, fungal, and parasitic causes should also be considered. As the CD4 count drops less than 200 cells/µL these infections become more common, and microsporidia, cryptosporidia, CMV, and *Mycobacterium avium-Mycobacterium intracellulare* may be the culprit.[46]

Highly Active Antiretroviral Therapy

The most common GI side effects of antiretroviral drug are nausea, vomiting, and diarrhea.[47]

Nevirapine may cause drug-related hepatitis and transaminitis; this occurs more often in patients with higher CD4 counts (>250 cells/mL in women and > 400 cells/mL in men).[48] The toxicity of nevirapine is associated with early hypersensitivity reactions, which can cause fulminant hepatitis with later onset of direct drug-related hepatotoxicity.[49] Tipranavir can cause severe hepatitis as well.[50] Atazanavir and indinavir have been noted to cause a Gilbert disease-like elevation in indirect bilirubin in nearly half of the patients.[51] As with Gilbert disease, this elevation is benign, and this occurs due to the inhibition of UGT1A1 and is not associated with other hepatic abnormalities.[52,53]

Didanosine, stavudine, and zidovudine can cause pancreatitis that is often seen in conjunction with a lactic acidosis.[51] Lopinavir/ritonavir can cause potentially fatal pancreatitis as well.[50]

Kaposi Sarcoma

Kaposi sarcoma (KS) accounts for 60% of overall malignancies and 40% of GI malignancies in patients with AIDS.[54] KS is caused by human herpesvirus 8. The most common GI sites include the stomach, duodenum, and biliary tract.[55] The jejunum, ileum, and large bowel are rarely involved. Approximately half of these cases of GI KS have associated skin lesions. GI involvement of KS can be found incidentally on endoscopy with up to 80% of lesions occurring without clinical symptoms.[55] Symptomatic presentation of GI KS is nonspecific and includes nausea, vomiting, anorexia, abdominal pain, diarrhea, and lower GI bleeding. Intussusception, obstruction, and perforation are possible complications of KS.[54] Early detection of GI KS is often difficult because symptoms often present later in the disease process. Particular at-risk populations include patients with CD4 count less than 100 cells/uL, patients with high viral load, those with cutaneous KS, and men who have sex with men.[56] Clinical suspicion should prompt endoscopy with biopsy and histologic testing for definitive diagnosis.[57,58]

A list of potential causes of abdominal pain in the patient with HIV/AIDS can be found in **Fig. 1**.

DIAGNOSTICS

Given the breadth of diagnostic possibilities in this special patient population, emergency physicians should pursue a broad diagnostic workup. A complete blood cell count with differential, comprehensive metabolic panel, lipase, pregnancy test for females, and urinalysis provides the beginning of this broad approach, with additional studies added on as needed based on the differential diagnosis. In the setting of diarrhea, stool studies including cultures and C difficile toxin testing may be beneficial. Imaging should focus on liberal use of cross-sectional imaging with computed tomography, with the addition of ultrasonography and magnetic resonance imaging as needed.

THERAPEUTICS

Treatment of patients with abdominal pain largely depends on the underlying cause. However, while workup is still ongoing and cause is unknown, the focus should rest on the patient-centered measure of pain control, as well as control of associated symptoms, such as nausea and vomiting. As most patients with abdominal pain should be kept nil per os (NPO) before definitive diagnosis, patients may benefit from intravenous fluid resuscitation or initiation of maintenance fluids if the NPO status is expected to be for an extended amount of time. Early administration of antibiotics should be considered for immunocompromised patients with any signs of infection, such as fever, hypotension, or altered mental status. Suspicion for structural abnormalities, such as obstruction, intussusception, or perforation, should prompt early surgical consultation. Suspicion for GVHD or PTLD should be discussed with the patient's transplant care team to coordinate a specific plan of care.

DISPOSITION

Care should be taken in determining the disposition of immunocompromised patients with abdominal pain. With a clear diagnosis requiring surgical treatment or the need for inpatient monitoring, patients can be swiftly admitted to an appropriate facility. Patients with structural abnormalities will require transfer to a hospital with surgical capabilities if this is not available at the presenting hospital. Treatment of posttransplant patients will often require transfer to their primary transplant center or close coordination with their transplant team if admission is not required. A more difficult situation arises when the diagnosis is uncertain and the patient continues to have symptoms. Low-risk, immunocompetent patients may be able to monitor themselves at home and return for a repeat abdominal examination, whereas caution should be exercised with immunocompromised patients. The increased risk of rapid deterioration of these patients limits the safety of at-home observation. These patients may require admission or observation for further advanced studies or serial abdominal examinations, even in the absence of a definitive diagnosis.

SUMMARY

Evaluation of abdominal pain in the immunocompromised patient requires a careful attention to detail and a thorough evaluation. After identifying immunocompromise based on congenital immunodeficiencies, malignancy, hematopoietic stem cell transplant, SOT, or HIV/AIDS, a targeted differential diagnosis may be considered. This differential will guide laboratory test ordering and imaging evaluation, as well as possible therapeutics to treat the underlying cause of the patient's pain. Despite the cause, conservative disposition strategies should be used in these high-risk individuals.

CLINICS CARE POINTS

- A careful history should be taken to identify patients with congenital, acquired, and medication-induced immunodeficiencies.

- Classic physical examination findings of serious abdominal pathologic condition may be absent in immunocompromised patients despite the presence of significant abnormalities.

- A differential diagnosis should be constructed by considering the patient's cause of immunocompromise, as well as the most likely emergencies associated with their underlying condition or medication.

- Laboratory testing should be broad, and cross-sectional imaging should be liberally used.

- A more conservative approach regarding disposition is prudent in this high-risk group.

DISCLOSURE

The authors have nothing to disclose.

REFERENCES

1. Cooper MA, Pommering TL, Korányi K. Primary immunodeficiencies. Am Fam Physician 2003;68(10):2001–8.
2. Amaya-Uribe L, Rojas M, Azizi G, et al. Primary immunodeficiency and autoimmunity: a comprehensive review. J Autoimmun 2019;99:52–72.
3. Jung A, Paauw D. Diagnosing HIV-related disease using the CD4 count as a guide. J Gen Intern Med 1998;13(2):131–6.
4. Obirikorang C, Quaye L, Acheampong I. Total lymphocyte count as a surrogate marker for CD4 count in resource-limited settings. BMC Infect Dis 2012;12:128.
5. Shapiro NI, Karras DJ, Leech SH, et al. Absolute lymphocyte count as a predictor of CD4 count. Ann Emerg Med 1998;32:323–8.
6. Chinen J, Shearer W. Secondary immunodeficiencies, including HIV infection. J Allergy Clin Immunol 2010;125:S195–203.
7. Berbudi A, Rahmadika N, Tjahjadi A, et al. Type 2 diabetes and its impact on the immune system. Curr Diabetes Rev 2020;16(5):442–9.
8. Cohen G. Immune dysfunction in uremia 2020. Toxins (Basel) 2020;12(7):439.
9. Bourke C, Berkley J, Prendergast A. Immune dysfunction as a cause and consequence of malnutrition. Trends Immunol 2016;37(6):386–98.
10. Fávaro-Moreira N, Krausch-Hofmann S, Matthys C, et al. Risk factors for malnutrition in older adults: a systematic review of the literature based on longitudinal data. Adv Nutr 2016;7(3):507–22.
11. Postow M, Callahan M, Wolchok J. Immune checkpoint blockade in cancer therapy. J Clin Oncol 2015;33(17):1974–82.
12. Del Castillo M, Romero F, Argüello E, et al. The spectrum of serious infections among patients receiving immune checkpoint blockade for the treatment of melanoma. Clin Infect Dis 2016;63(11):1490–3.

13. Axelrod D, Naik A, Schnitzler M, et al. National variation in use of immunosuppression for kidney transplantation: a call for evidence-based regimen selection. Am J Transpl 2016;16(8):2453–62.
14. Focosi D, Maggi F, Pistello M, et al. Immunosuppressive monoclonal antibodies: current and next generation. Clin Microbiol Infect 2011;17(12):1759–68.
15. Rosenfeld P, Brown D, Heier J, et al. Ranibizumab for neovascular age-related macular degeneration. N Engl J Med 2006;355(14):1419–31.
16. Goldburg S, Strober B, Payette M. Hidradenitis suppurativa: Current and emerging treatments. J Am Acad Dermatol 2020;82(5):1061–82.
17. Normansell R, Walker S, Milan SJ, et al. Omalizumab for asthma in adults and children. Cochrane Database Syst Rev 2014;(1):CD003559.
18. Chong L, Piromchai P, Sharp S, et al. Biologics for chronic rhinosinusitis. Cochrane Database Syst Rev 2021;3(3):CD013513.
19. Lindorfer M, Pawluczkowycz A, Peek E, et al. A novel approach to preventing the hemolysis of paroxysmal nocturnal hemoglobinuria: both complement-mediated cytolysis and C3 deposition are blocked by a monoclonal antibody specific for the alternative pathway of complement. Blood 2010;115(11):2283–91.
20. Marovich M, Mascola J, Cohen M. Monoclonal Antibodies for Prevention and Treatment of COVID-19. JAMA 2020;324(2):131–2.
21. Tomblyn M, Chiller T, Einsele H, et al. Guidelines for preventing infectious complications among hematopoietic cell transplantation recipients: a global perspective. Biol Blood Marrow Transpl 2009;15(10):1143–238.
22. Agarwal S, Cunningham-Rundles C. Gastrointestinal manifestations and complications of primary immunodeficiency disorders. Immunol Allergy Clin North Am 2019;39(1):81–94.
23. Touchefeu Y. Systematic review: the role of the gut microbiota in chemotherapy- or radiation-induced gastrointestinal mucositis – current evidence and potential clinical applications. Aliment Pharmacol Ther 2014;49(5):409–21.
24. Keefe D. Intestinal mucositis: mechanisms and management. Curr Opin Oncol 2007;19:323–7.
25. Elting LS, Cooksley C, Chambers M, et al. The burdens of cancer therapy. Clinical and economic outcomes of chemotherapy-induced mucositis. Cancer 2003;98:1531–9.
26. Lebon D, Biard L, Buyse S, et al. Gastrointestinal emergencies in critically ill cancer patients. J Crit Care 2017;40:69–75.
27. Cunningham S, Fakhry K, Bass B, et al. Neutropenic enterocolitis in adults: case series and review of the literature. Dig Dis Sci 2005;50:215–20.
28. Nesher L, Rolston K. Neutropenic enterocolitis, a growing concern in the era of widespread use of aggressive chemotherapy. Clin Infect Dis 2013;56:711–7.
29. Rodrigues F, Dasilva G, Wexner SD. Neutropenic enterocolitis. World J Gastroenterol 2017;23(1):42–7.
30. Cartoni C, Dragoni F, Micozzi A, et al. Neutropenic enterocolitis in patients with acute leukemia: prognostic significance of bowel wall thickening detected by ultrasonography. J Clin Oncol 2001;19(3):756–61.
31. Tuca A, Guell E, Martinez-Losada E, et al. Malignant bowel obstruction in advanced cancer patients: epidemiology, management, and factors influencing spontaneous resolution. Cancer Manag Res 2012;4:159–69.
32. Gonzalez-Hernandea J, Garcia F. Cecal adenocarcinoma presenting as colonic intussusception in adulthood. Proc Bayl Univ Med Cen 2015;28(2):180–2.
33. Carden M, Little J. Emerging disease-modifying therapies for sickle cell disease. Haematologica 2019;104(9):1710–9.

34. Naymagon S, Naymagon L, Wong S, et al. Acute graft-versus-host disease of the gut: considerations for the gastroenterologist. Nat Rev Gastroenterol Hepatol 2017;14(12):711–26.
35. Schlick K, Grundbichler M, Auberger J, et al. Cytomegalovirus reactivation and its clinical impact in patients with solid tumors. Infect Agent Cancer 2015;10:45.
36. Sen A, Callisen H, Libricz S, et al. Complications of solid organ transplantation: cardiovascular, neurologic, renal, and gastrointestinal. Crit Care Clin 2019; 35(1):169–86.
37. Mori T, Mori S, Kanda Y, et al. Clinical significance of cytomegalovirus antigenemia in the prediction and diagnosis of CMV gastrointestinal disease after allogenic hematopoietic stem cell transplantation. Bone Marrow Transpl 2004; 33(4):431–43.
38. Ison M. Editorial commentary: diagnosis of gastrointestinal cytomegalovirus infections: an imperfect science. Clin Infect Dis 2013;57(11):1560–1.
39. Graham SM, Flowers JL, Schweitzer E, et al. Opportunistic upper gastrointestinal infection in transplant recipients. Surg Endosc 1995;9(2):146–50.
40. Cimino F, Snyder K. Primary care of the solid organ transplant patient. Am Fam Physician 2016;93(3):203–10.
41. Larson A, Issaka R, Hockenbery D. Gastrointestinal and hepatic complications of solid organ and hematopoietic cell transplantation. In: Feldman M, Friedman S, Brandt L, editors. Sleisinger and Fordtran's gastrointestinal and liver disease. 11th edition. Elsevier; 2020. p. 510–31.
42. Helderman J, Goral S. Gastrointestinal complications of transplant immunosuppression. J Am Soc Nephrol 2002;12(1):277–87.
43. Opelz G, Döhler B. Lymphomas after solid organ transplantation: a collaborative transplant study report. Am J Transpl 2004;4(2):222–30.
44. Taylor A, Marcus R, Bradley J. Post-transplant lymphoproliferative disorders (PTLD) after solid organ transplantation. Crit Rev Oncol Hematol 2005;56(1): 155–67.
45. Burns D, Crawford D. Epstein-Barr virus-specific cytotoxic T-lymphocytes for adoptive immunotherapy of post-transplant lymphoproliferative disease. Blood Rev 2004;18(3):193–209.
46. Collini P, Kuijper E, Dockrell D. Clostridium difficile infection in patients with HIV/ AIDS. Curr HIV/AIDS Rep 2013;10:273–82.
47. Sharpstone D, Gazzard B. Gastrointestinal manifestations of HIV. Lancet 1996; 348(9024):379–83.
48. Hall VP. Common gastrointestinal complications associated with human immunodeficiency Virus/AIDS: an overview. Crit Care Nurs Clin North Am 2018;30(1): 101–7.
49. Gulick R. Antiretroviral therapy for human immunodeficiency virus and acquired immunodeficiency syndrome. In: Goldman L, Schafer A, editors. Goldman-cecil medicine. 25th edition. Philadelphia: Elsevier; 2016. p. 2255–60.
50. Mbougua J, Laurent C, Kouanfack C, et al. Hepatotoxicity and effectiveness of a nevirapine-based antiretroviral therapy in HIV-infected patients without viral hepatitis B or C infection in camerron. BMC Public Health 2010;10:105.
51. Reust C. Common adverse effects of antiretroviral therapy for HIV disease. Am Fam Physician 2011;83(12):1443–51.
52. Venkat A, Piontkowsky D, Cooney R, et al. Care of the HIV-positive patient in the emergency department in the era of highly active antiretroviral therapy. Ann Emer Med 2008;52(3):274–85.

53. Neuman M, Schnieder M, Nanau R, et al. HIV-antiretroviral therapy induced liver, gastrointestinal, and pancreatic injury. Int J Hepatol 2012;2012:1–23.
54. Zucker S, Qin X, Rouster S, et al. Mechanism of indinavir-induced hyperbilirubinemia. Proc Natl Acad Sci U S A 2001;98(22):12671–6.
55. Nidimusili A, Eisa N, Shaheen K. Gastrointestinal Kaposi's sarcoma presenting as ileocolic intussusception. N Am J Med Sci 2013;5(11):666–8.
56. Parente F, Cernuschi M, Orlando G, et al. Kaposi's sarcoma and AIDS: frequency of gastrointestinal involvement and its effect on survival. A prospective study in a heterogeneous population. Scand J Gastroenterol 1991;26(10):1007–12.
57. Nagata N, Shimbo T, Yazaki H, et al. Predictive clinical factors in the diagnosis of gastrointestinal Kaposi's sarcoma and its endoscopic severity. PLoS One 2012; 7(11):e46967.
58. Lee AJ, Brenner L, Mourad B, et al. Gastrointestinal Kaposi's sarcoma: Case report and review of the literature. World J Gastrointest Pharmacol Ther 2015; 6(3):89–95.

Chronic Drug Use and Abdominal Pain

Alexis L. Cates, DO[a],*, Brenna Farmer, MD, MBA, MS[b,1]

KEYWORDS

- Alcohol use disorder • Opioid use disorder • Gastrointestinal emergencies
- Hepatotoxicity • Chronic drug use

KEY POINTS

- Alcohol use disorder contributes to emergent pathology throughout the gastrointestinal tract and liver.
- Chronic opioid use contributes to often unrelenting constipation.
- Building a rapport with patients who have substance use disorders is important to gain the history and insight needed to guide your diagnostic differential.

INTRODUCTION

It is well known that abdominal pain and related complaints are among the top reasons for Emergency Department (ED) visits. The National Hospital Ambulatory Medical Care Survey (NHAMCS) in 2017 noted that injury and poisonings also make up a significant percentage, 18.9%, of the primary diagnoses for ED visits. Alcohol use disorder and substance use disorder are associated with 3.1% and 5.8% of all ED visits, respectively.[1] There is overlap in these diagnoses, and it is not surprising patients present with a combination of these diagnoses. In this article, we discuss a general approach to abdominal pain in patients with chronic drug and alcohol use disorders with an emphasis on an expanded diagnostic differential. Several substance-specific diagnoses and therapeutic options for the management of chronic abdominal pain in patients with substance use disorders are highlighted.

APPROACH

The general approach to abdominal pain in a patient with chronic drug use includes a detailed history, review of systems, medications, allergies, and an in-depth discussion

[a] Division of Medical Toxicology, Department of Emergency Medicine, Einstein Healthcare Network, Korman B-14, 5501 Old York Road, Philadelphia, PA 19141, USA; [b] Quality and Patient Safety, Department of Emergency Medicine, Weill Cornell Medicine, New York Presbyterian/Lower Manhattan Hospital Emergency Department
[1] Present address: Department of Emergency Medicine, 525 E 68th St., New York, NY 10065, USA.
* Corresponding author.
E-mail address: catesale@einstein.edu

Emerg Med Clin N Am 39 (2021) 821–837
https://doi.org/10.1016/j.emc.2021.07.006
0733-8627/21/© 2021 Elsevier Inc. All rights reserved.

of social history and substance use. The substance use history should include types of substances used and frequency of use, routes of exposure, methods in which the patient obtains the substance, and any recent changes to use patterns. A detailed physical examination as guided by the history should follow.

A broad list of differential diagnoses should be developed based on the history and physical examination. Certain substance use may add a specific diagnosis to the differential. Testing can then be tailored to the clinician's suspicions.

General laboratory testing in patients with substance use concerns may include complete metabolic panel, complete blood count, serum acetaminophen and salicylate levels (as common coingestants), ethanol level, serum osmolality, urinalysis, and pregnancy testing. Occasionally, if the patient's presentation lends concern for specific organ dysfunction, labs such as amylase and/or lipase, troponin, urine and blood cultures, viral hepatitis panels and testing for commonly transmitted infections may be considered.

A urine drug screen may be useful to determine previous exposure to a particular drug of abuse such as cocaine, tetrahydrocannabinol (THC), or opioids. It is not helpful for diagnosing acute intoxication or withdrawal, nor is it inclusive of all drug exposures. Urine immunoassays may only include opiates or the compounds that include or metabolize to morphine or codeine. Therefore, there is limited utility in a patient that may have been exposed to a semisynthetic or synthetic opioid such as methadone, oxycodone, or fentanyl. Some laboratories may have the ability to screen for specific opioids such as fentanyl, 6-monoacetylmorphine (the metabolite of heroin), tramadol, methadone, and buprenorphine or obtain more specific testing via gas chromatography and mass spectrometry.[2]

In addition to laboratory testing, imaging studies can greatly increase diagnostic accuracy. Plain radiographs, ultrasonography, computed tomography (CT), and or MRI may be helpful depending on the differential diagnosis and is discussed below with specific substances.

CLINICAL RELEVANCE

There are numerous gastrointestinal manifestations of chronic alcohol and drug use. Although the NHAMCS survey was limited and diagnoses potentially underreported, alcohol-related disorders accounted for 0.8% and opioid-related disorders reported for 0.1% of all diagnoses made in the ED setting.[1] The use of both substances likely accounts for abdominal pain due to disorders of the gastrointestinal tract, as well as abdominal pain due to disorders of the cardiovascular and genitourinary systems. The focus of this article will be on frequently encountered substances of abuse and associated common gastrointestinal pathologies, as well as emergent evaluation and pertinent diagnostics. The most detailed discussion will occur with ethanol and opioids, given the evidence supporting abdominal complaints with chronic use.

ETHANOL

Ethanol, more commonly called "alcohol," is one of the most used substances in the world. Excessive alcohol use and subsequent damage to the gastrointestinal tract are vast. As the site of alcohol absorption, the gastrointestinal tract can be negatively affected by numerous metabolic and functional changes and has been extensively researched.[3] The pathology can vary widely, from simple gastritis to esophageal varices and from oral lesions to numerous cancers.

Esophagus and Stomach

Chronic alcohol use may lead to a variety of disorders in the esophagus and stomach. In the acute period following alcohol consumption, there may be an increase in symptoms of gastroesophageal reflux (GERD). GERD symptoms can lead to vomiting and potentially Mallory-Weiss syndrome.[4] Esophageal bleeding may also be indicative of esophageal varices, as a complication of portal venous hypertension in patients with cirrhosis. Persistent vomiting and increased pressure in the portal venous system could lead to variceal rupture, a potentially fatal complication producing significant upper gastrointestinal hemorrhage.[5] Obtaining complete blood counts, hepatic panels, and coagulation studies are critical in defining severity of disease. In addition, type and screen with crossmatching of blood is necessary to allow for blood product replacement during resuscitation. Advanced diagnostic and therapeutic interventions such as esophagogastroduodenoscopy are often indicated while resuscitative efforts continue.

Boerhaave's syndrome, a tear in the esophageal mucosa leading to complete spontaneous rupture, can be associated with chronic alcohol use. It occurs following a sudden increase in intra-esophageal pressure due to persistent vomiting. Vomiting, chest pain, and subcutaneous emphysema are classic findings.[6] Chest x-rays cannot be used to exclude the diagnosis but may identify abnormalities such as subcutaneous or mediastinal emphysema, mediastinal widening, or associated pleural effusion concerning for this diagnosis. Advanced imaging such as a contrast-enhanced CT scan of the chest, abdomen, and pelvis are more specific. Significant complications requiring surgical intervention may occur, so early surgical consultation is recommended.

Inflammation along the stomach lining, or gastritis, may also cause hemorrhage due to ulceration. There is a known association between alcohol use and the development of active *Helicobacter pylori* infection, as well, which can contribute to ongoing discomfort.[7] Peptic ulcer disease may be multifactorial and is not likely to be directly associated with an increase in alcohol consumption.[8]

Pancreas

Pancreatic disease is commonly associated with morbidity and mortality due to chronic alcohol use. Gallstones and excessive alcohol use are most commonly associated with acute pancreatitis in Western societies, although the amount to which either contributes varies among geographic regions and alcohol consumption patterns.[4] Two explanations of the mechanism involved include the premature activation of pancreatic enzymes within the acinar cell (auto-digestion) and organelle dysfunction leading to abnormal secretion of digestive enzymes.[4,9]

Patients may present with reported prior acute pancreatitis and a history of significant alcohol use. Mild symptoms of abdominal discomfort with nausea and vomiting can occur, whereas severe cases may develop multi-organ dysfunction, infection, and complications such as abscesses, pseudocysts, or necrosis. There is often abdominal tenderness, particularly in the upper abdomen and epigastric region. Diagnosis of acute pancreatitis is made by the presence of at least two of the following: significant upper abdominal pain typically radiating to the back, serum lipase or amylase levels that are at least three times the upper limit of normal, or findings on advanced imaging such as contrast-enhanced CT of the abdomen.[9,10] Other causes of acute pancreatitis should be excluded by history, physical examination, laboratory results, advanced imaging, and procedures such as endoscopic retrograde cholangiopancreatography as indicated.[4]

Chronic pancreatitis is characterized by often irreversible fibrosis and inflammation, atrophy, calcifications, dysplasia, exocrine or endocrine insufficiency, and chronic abdominal pain. Although there are multiple potential causes for chronic pancreatitis (eg, hypertriglyceridemia and hyperparathyroidism), the diagnosis is most commonly associated with excessive alcohol use in 75% of cases.[4,11] A linear dose–response relationship with increasing daily alcohol intake is associated with development of chronic pancreatitis.[12] Other risk factors include concomitant use of smoking tobacco and certain genetic factors.[4] Patients often present with severe upper abdominal pain that radiates to the back, increasing with meals and subsequently leading to decreased appetite. Patients may also present with steatorrhea, new-onset diabetes, and significant weight loss.

Chronic pancreatitis is primarily a clinical diagnosis; however, owing to complications such as pseudocyst formations, biliary obstructions, pseudoaneurysms, and cancer, imaging such as contrast-enhanced CT or MRI is often obtained. Amylase and lipase levels may be normal as the disease progresses and more fibrotic tissue replaces pancreatic parenchyma.[13]

Liver

Alcoholic liver disease (ALD) is one of the major causes of chronic liver disease in the United States. The term covers a spectrum of hepatic disorders, from steatosis and hepatitis to irreversible alcoholic cirrhosis. Several factors may play a role in the development of ALD, including gender, obesity, and metabolic, genetic, environmental, and immunologic factors. However, the largest risk factor is the quantity and duration of alcohol use, with an increase of either correlating with disease development.[14] ALD and continued use may synergistically impair hepatic function with the presence of other hepatotoxins such as acetaminophen, infections such as hepatitis C and human immunodeficiency virus, and nutritional impairments.[15,16]

Alcohol itself is a hepatotoxin. The end products of alcohol metabolism, such as acetaldehyde, damage the liver by triggering inflammation and fibrogenesis.[16] A spectrum of clinical syndromes can occur, ranging from asymptomatic illness to end-stage liver disease. A patient with hepatic steatosis may present with right upper quadrant discomfort, nausea, vomiting, and anorexia.[15] The liver may be normal or enlarged in size. A patient with alcoholic hepatitis may present with jaundice, anorexia, right upper quadrant pain, fever, ascites, and enlarged liver. These symptoms may be more insidious when compared with a viral or toxin-mediated hepatitis. More severe cases of alcoholic cirrhosis may feature hepatic encephalopathy and synthetic liver dysfunction, reflecting impending hepatic failure.[15]

Alcoholic cirrhosis may lead to hepatorenal syndrome, of which the complicated pathophysiology is beyond the scope of this article. However, this syndrome may be identified on recognition of a patient in extremis with oliguria and an insidious increase in serum creatinine, thought to be related to renal vasoconstriction and associated fulminant liver failure.[17] Despite adequate resuscitation and removal of any potentially nephrotoxic or hepatotoxic xenobiotics to explain the clinical presentation, patients with this syndrome have a poor prognosis and may ultimately require liver transplantation.[17]

Although a history of excessive alcohol use may indicate ALD and related complications, other causes of hepatobiliary disease and liver failure should be considered. Diagnostic imaging dedicated to the hepatobiliary system may be beneficial in this delineation, including but not limited to abdominal ultrasonography. Laboratory abnormalities seen with ALD may include thrombocytopenia, anemia, elevated liver transaminases (often   a   greater   increase   in   aspartate   aminotransferase), hypoalbuminemia, hyperbilirubinemia, elevated gamma-glutamyl transpeptidase (GGTP), elevated prothrombin time, and international normalized ratio (INR) and possible renal dysfunction or electrolyte abnormalities.[14] A viral hepatitis panel may also be beneficial in ruling out concomitant acute or chronic viral etiologies.

Small Intestine, Large Intestine, and Rectum

Chronic alcohol use can lead to diarrhea due to impaired gut motility, permeability, nutritional disorders, and impaired absorption of critical vitamins and nutrients.[4] Associated folate deficiency due to reduced intake and impaired liver function can further malabsorption.[18] Although alcohol is not likely to directly transit through the gut to the large intestine, there may be indirect mucosal damage from significant inflammatory responses resulting in the loss of mucosal integrity and contributing to impaired permeability.[16] Toxic metabolites of alcohol such as acetaldehyde can contribute to carcinogenesis.[16] Lastly, colonic varices due to portal hypertension can occur, and bleeding from hemorrhoids may be increased.[4]

Miscellaneous Effects

Chronic use of alcohol can contribute to a variety of other pathologies not mentioned here, due to the limitations of this article. This does not imply a lack of importance, however. Many of these other pathologies may involve abdominal pain as one of the presenting symptoms.

Alcoholic ketoacidosis (AKA) can be seen in patients with chronic ethanol use due to the cessation of adequate nutrition during a "binge" drinking episode or due to nausea, vomiting, and abdominal pain from related gastritis, hepatitis, pancreatitis, or other illness.[19] Findings will include significant dehydration, nausea, vomiting, abdominal discomfort, tachycardia, tachypnea, and presence of ketoacids, mainly in the form of beta-hydroxybutyrate.[20] Alcohol withdrawal following an abrupt cessation or significant decline in use may also present with gastrointestinal and central nervous system complaints and may contribute to AKA.

Additionally, alcohol is a cocarcinogen, increasing cancer risk of those patients exposed to another carcinogen. In a compilation of meta-analyses, chronic alcohol use is associated with increased risk of gastrointestinal carcinogenesis, including cancers of the tongue, mouth, pharynx, esophagus, stomach, pancreas, colon, and liver.[21]

Therapeutic Options

Initial resuscitation would include usual care of airway management, placement of intravenous lines, volume resuscitation, glucose administration, and vitamin and electrolyte supplementation as needed. Blood products would be indicated in massive gastrointestinal hemorrhage. Pain control in the form of parenteral opioids or other non-opioid analgesics may be warranted, depending on the suspected diagnosis. Monitoring patients for alcohol withdrawal and treating as needed can mitigate in-hospital comorbid conditions. Controlled cessation of alcohol use and therapeutic options therein should be discussed. Molecular Adsorbent Recirculating System (MARS), essentially a liver replacement therapy, has been used in patients with liver failure.[22]

OPIOIDS

Opioid agonists have been used as pharmacotherapy for acute or chronic pain for centuries.[23] Unfortunately, the addicting effects of opioids have led to abuse of both prescription and illicit opioids with an increasing group of patients meeting criteria for opioid use disorder (OUD).[a]

In 2016, there were 1.9 million American adults with OUD with approximately 360,000 persons enrolled in a federally licensed treatment program.[24] It is not uncommon for the gastrointestinal effects associated with opioids to lead patients to seek medical care.

Opioids commonly decrease gastrointestinal motility with symptoms manifesting as constipation, bloating, early satiety, and pain leading to bowel dysfunction with blockade of peristalsis and an overall decrease in intestinal fluids.[4] In contrast, opioid withdrawal results in nausea, vomiting, diarrhea, and abdominal cramping. The following is a discussion of common gastrointestinal complaints related to opioid use.

Narcotic Bowel Syndrome

Narcotic bowel syndrome describes the progressive increase of colicky abdominal pain with continued or increased use of opioids.[b]

One of the perpetuating factors is likely related to the hyperalgesia effects of opioids, although exact molecular mechanisms are poorly understood.[25] Increasing doses of opioids in response to pain enhance adverse effects on pain sensation and ultimately delays gastrointestinal motility.[4] Ideal treatment includes a biopsychosocial approach of appropriate opioid weaning, prevention or reduction of opioid withdrawal symptoms, aggressive bowel regimen, alternative therapies for pain control, and behavioral health intervention.

If obtaining an abdominal plain film, be mindful that, in instances of presumed narcotic bowel syndrome, there may be evidence of a partial intestinal obstruction, which is more likely due to adynamic ileus or a pseudo-obstruction.[26] There may also be a large amount of retained fecal matter. In instances where more advanced imaging would be needed, a contrast-enhanced CT of the abdomen and pelvis may be beneficial.

Motility Disorders

Motility disorders such as opioid-induced constipation (OIC) and esophageal motility disorders occur from chronic opioid use.

OIC may present immediately or gradually over time. Opioid-replacement therapies such as methadone and buprenorphine have also been associated with OIC.[27] Norbuprenorphine, the active metabolite of buprenorphine, may play more of a role as the opioid receptor agonist while buprenorphine itself has a higher risk of OIC.[28]

OIC is due to inhibition of gastric emptying or inhibition of peristalsis resulting in delayed absorption of medications and increased absorption of fluid, hardening of stool, and ultimately constipation.[29] Other gastrointestinal symptoms may develop such as nausea, vomiting, and bloating.

The effects of opioids on esophageal motility have been evaluated in small studies with variable results.[30] Chronic use of opioids may lead to dysphagia or GERD due to impairment at lower esophageal sphincter and potentially esophagogastric junction outflow obstruction.[31] A large retrospective study of chronic opioid users noted

---

[a] Opioid Use Disorder (OUD): Defined by the Diagnostic and Statistical Manual of Mental Disorders, Fifth Edition (DSM-5) as a problematic pattern of opioid use leading to clinically significant impairment or distress.

[b] Although the term "narcotic" is not favored when describing opioids, this term has been widely recognized in the literature in the setting of "narcotic bowel syndrome," and so it is used in this article.

esophageal dysmotility with increased esophagogastric junction outflow obstruction and esophageal spasticity within 24 hours of use.[30]

Hepatic Disease Related to Opioid Use

Currently, there are no evidence-based studies demonstrating hepatotoxicity from pure opioid agonists. One case report from 2008 identified suspected cholestatic hepatitis, diagnosed via liver biopsy, thought to be related to oxycodone use.[32]

Patients who chronically use or misuse opioids may expose themselves to opioid combination products, such as oxycodone with acetaminophen. Unfortunately, the combination with acetaminophen has been linked to acute liver failure, mostly from unintentional overdose with acetaminophen.[33] Many patients may not be aware of the acetaminophen coproduct and could potentially take more than is prescribed or use the product illicitly. Some may take additional acetaminophen or other hepatotoxic medications.

Hepatic disease such as hepatitis B and C related to injection opioid use could be a cause of nausea, vomiting, abdominal pain, and jaundice. In particular, the number of hepatitis C infections has risen dramatically since 2009 correlating with injection opioid use patterns.[34] Unsafe injecting practices contribute substantially to these rising infections.[35] Although specific treatment is not likely to be initiated in the emergency setting, diagnosis and arranging outpatient follow-up is important. If left untreated, continued transmission to others is possible and places further strain on the health care system.

Opioid Withdrawal

Depending on the opioid, a patient can experience symptoms of opioid withdrawal with variation in onset after a sudden reduction in use or abstinence. It may also occur when a partial agonist or antagonist is introduced in the presence of agonists bound to the mu opioid receptors. Opioid withdrawal symptoms are complex and beyond the scope of this article, except for mention of gastrointestinal symptoms such as nausea, vomiting, abdominal cramping, and diarrhea. These symptoms are due to the presence of opioid receptors in the gastrointestinal tract. Although opioid withdrawal is not likely to result in severe morbidity or mortality directly, it can cause significant discomfort and be temporarily disabling. Persistent vomiting or diarrhea can lead to fluid and electrolyte derangements with acute kidney injury. Poorly treated opioid withdrawal may result in decreased tolerance over time, such that if the patient seeks opioid agonist use again, a significant overdose may occur and indirectly increase morbidity and mortality.

Treatment of the gastrointestinal symptoms of opioid withdrawal is often guided by supportive care. Fluid resuscitation, electrolyte replacement, and antiemetics may be needed. Initiation of medication-assisted treatment (MAT) with medications such as buprenorphine, methadone, or naltrexone will also likely provide relief of these symptoms. A clinical opioid withdrawal scale can assess for severity of opioid withdrawal symptoms and assist in determination of appropriate intervention with MAT in combination with symptomatic management.

Therapeutic Options

The approach for patients with OUD can begin with an evaluation for potential weaning of opioid use as much as possible. If this is not feasible, a variety of other therapeutics may be employed, depending on the symptoms.

Conservative measures to relieve opioid-induced bowel dysfunction may be attempted with increased fluid intake, dietary fiber supplementation, and osmotic laxatives.[36] For more complicated cases or those that do not respond to conservative measures, numerous pharmaceutical interventions can be considered.

Patients who use opioids for pain control long-term may find some benefit in oral preparations of opioid agonists with naloxone for improved bowel function and analgesia without the effects of opioid withdrawal.[37-39] Preparations such as the long-acting mu opioid antagonist methylnaltrexone and naloxegol do not penetrate the blood brain barrier, but rather exhibit their activity peripherally to counteract full opioid agonists' effect on the gut.[40] OIC relief is often slow and full resolution is difficult. A summary of common pharmaceutical treatments are found in **Table 1**.

In patients with illicit use, MAT would be ideal, leading them away from opioid misuse to a regulated and supervised treatment program. This treatment involves a combination of biopsychosocial approaches plus office-based pharmacotherapy, such as buprenorphine, buprenorphine/naloxone combination products, methadone or naltrexone (**Table 2**). Unfortunately, there is still a high prevalence of OIC in patients treated with MAT, in particular methadone and buprenorphine.[41] In these patients, the preferred treatment is a supportive bowel regimen with increased fluid, fiber intake, and osmotic laxatives as needed.

Patients with acute opioid withdrawal will also present to the ED with gastrointestinal distress; treatment should include symptomatic and supportive care (**Table 3**). Opioid replacement therapy can also be initiated depending on the circumstances, as shown in **Table 2**. Maintenance therapy is represented by one of the following: gradual cessation of an opioid agonist, use of a partial mu-opioid agonist, or use of an opioid antagonist as maintenance.[42] The more uncomfortable symptomatology that patients experience are the gastrointestinal symptoms and may lead the patient to further misuse opioid agonists to treat their symptoms.[24] Occasionally, patients with OUD and concomitant painful medical or surgical pathology will require short-acting opioid agonists for pain control and withdrawal symptoms. Appropriate tapering to abstinence or MAT is worth consideration following resolution of said pathology.

AMPHETAMINES

Although there are select derivatives approved for medicinal use, amphetamines are also commonly drugs of abuse. Users seek the central stimulatory effects and effects caused by an increase in neurotransmission of dopamine, norepinephrine, and serotonin.[43] Amphetamines are addicting, and long-term effects are still under evaluation.[44] In relation to the gastrointestinal tract, certain amphetamines have been associated with gut ischemia, hepatotoxicity, and liver failure.

Numerous case reports describe significant intra-abdominal pathology secondary to poor organ perfusion in sympathomimetic and vasoconstrictive states due to amphetamine use. The accumulation of norepinephrine postsynaptically contributes to systemic hypertension, tachycardia, and local vasospasm or vasoconstriction leading to organ ischemia. Chronic use may exacerbate this effect, and fatalities have been reported.[45] Ischemic colitis, small bowel ischemia, gangrenous cholecystitis, ulcerations of the intestines, and perforated viscus are all reported.[45-50] Surgical consultation should be considered.

Significant hepatotoxicity, though rare, has been identified as a complication of the use of 3,4-methylenedioxymethamphetamine (MDMA, Ecstasy) and synthetic cathinones (bath salts), another sympathomimetic drug of abuse. Although hepatitis may result from the use of contaminated needles with viral hepatitis, there are also reports of direct hepatotoxicity.[51] Patients present with abdominal pain, systemic toxicity, and accompanying fulminant liver failure, or they with jaundice present days to weeks

Table 1
Opioid-induced constipation (OIC) treatment options

Medication/Mechanism of Action	Dosing/Routes/frequency	Indication	Caution
Docusate sodium (Surfactant laxative, stool softener)	50 mg - 300 mg daily or divided doses	Adults with constipation	Avoid with intestinal obstruction or risk for perforation Avoid concomitant use with mineral oil Avoid use >7 d
Methylnaltrexone (peripherally acting mu opioid antagonist)	12 mg SC daily OR 450 mg PO daily in AM	Adults with OIC and chronic non-cancer pain	Avoid with intestinal obstruction or risk for perforation Needs renal/hepatic adjustments
Naloxegol (peripherally acting mu opioid antagonist)	12.5 mg to 25 mg PO per day in the AM (1 h AC or 2 h PC)	Adults with OIC and chronic non-cancer pain	Do not administer with CYP3A4 inducers or inhibitors Avoid with intestinal obstruction or risk for perforation
Oxycodone-Naloxone (Combination mu opioid agonist and antagonist)	Initial dose 10 mg/5 mg tablet PO up to twice daily Not to exceed daily dose of 80 mg/40 mg (or 40 mg/20 mg twice daily)	Adults with chronic severe pain and OIC	Avoid with other opioid agonists Needs renal/hepatic adjustments
Polyethylene glycol (osmotic laxative)	17 g packet or large spoonful of oral powder in 4-8 oz of beverage (water) daily	Adults with constipation	Avoid with intestinal obstruction or risk for perforation Avoid with intestinal infection Avoid with concomitant use of stimulant laxatives Monitor electrolytes Avoid use >7 d Caution in renal impairment
Senna (intestinal irritant and stimulant)	15 mg PO once daily Not to exceed daily dose of 70–100 mg	Adults with constipation	Avoid with intestinal obstruction or risk for perforation Avoid use >7 d

[a]Options may include usual symptomatic and supportive care as with other similar conditions, or specific products to target mu opioid receptors of the gastrointestinal tract.

Table 2
Medication-assisted therapy for opioid use disorder (OUD)

Medication/Mechanism of Action	Dosing/Routes/Frequency	Indication	Caution
Buprenorphine *(Partial agonist at mu opioid receptor)*	*Dosing/Frequency:* varies depending on patient response. Typical initial dosing: 4 mg - 8 mg but can be as high as 16 mg - 32 mg. hen, 4 mg - 24 mg daily, divided into daily, twice daily or three times daily dosing. *Routes:* sublingual (disintegrating tab)	Maintenance in OUD. Monoproduct is therapy of choice for pregnant patients.	Precipitated withdrawal possible in presence of full mu opioid agonists. Has some value on illicit markets as monoproduct.
Buprenorphine/Naloxone *(partial agonist at mu opioid receptor with poorly bioavailable antagonist at mu opioid receptor when administered sublingually)*	*Dosing/Frequency:* varies depending on patient response. Typical initial dosing: 4 mg - 8 mg but can be as high as 16 mg - 32 mg. Then, 4 mg - 24 mg daily, divided into daily, twice daily or three times daily dosing. *Routes:* sublingual (disintegrating strip)	Maintenance in OUD.	Precipitated withdrawal possible in presence of full mu opioid agonists. Not indicated for pregnant patients due to potential for naloxone to cause withdrawal in fetus.
Methadone *(long-acting full agonist at mu opioid receptor)*	*Dosing/Frequency:* Varies depending on patient response. Initial daily dosing 30mg-40 mg. *Routes:* oral	Maintenance in OUD.	Strict rules on credentialing of distributing pharmacies; usually associated with a daily clinic. Caution with QTc prolongation and escalating doses.
Naltrexone *(long-acting antagonist at mu opioid receptor)*	*Dosing/Frequency:* Initial dose 25 mg then upwards to 50 mg daily in oral form. 380 mg every 4 wk in injection form. *Routes:* oral tab, intra-muscular	Maintenance in OUD.	May have loss of tolerance to opioids during a relapse period.

[a]Currently, buprenorphine prescriptions greater than 3 days (72 h) must be written by those with a waiver to their Drug Enforcement Administration (DEA) license. This is subject to change.

Table 3
Common medications[a] used for treatment of opioid withdrawal

Medication	Dosing/Route/ Frequency	Indication	Caution
Acetaminophen	650 mg PO every 4– 6 h, maximum 4 g/ d	Abdominal pain, myalgias	May contribute to hepatotoxicity
Clonidine	0.1 mg PO every 6– 8 h, maximum 1.2 mg/d	Anxiety, CNS hyperexcitation	May cause bradycardia and hypotension
Dicyclomine	20 mg IM or PO every 6 h	Abdominal cramping	
Ibuprofen	600 mg PO every 4– 6 h	Abdominal pain, myalgias	May cause gastritis
Loperamide	2–4 mg PO every every 6 h, maximum 16 mg/d	Diarrhea	May be misused, and in high doses may cause prolonged QTc interval
Metoclopramide	10 mg IV or PO every 6 h	Nausea, vomiting	
Ondansetron	4–8 mg IV or SL every 8 h	Nausea, vomiting	May cause prolonged QTc interval
Prochlorperazine	2.5 mg - 10 mg IV every 4 h, maximum 40 mg/d	Nausea, vomiting	

[a] These commonly used substances may be considered in the absence of other contraindications and in conjunction with opioid replacement therapy.

following the exposure potentially progressing to fulminant liver failure.[15] Patient history is key to differentiate from other causes. This disease process may be multifactorial, particularly when the patient may also suffer from hepatic dysfunction due to hyperthermia, hypovolemia resulting in poor organ perfusion, and rhabdomyolysis.[15] Treatment is largely supportive but may also include infusions such as N-acetylcysteine when drug-induced liver injury is suspected. Some cases may be fatal or lead to liver transplantation.[15]

CANNABINOIDS

Cannabinoids extracted from the plant *Cannabis sativa* have long been used for proposed medicinal properties in addition to euphoric effects. Although policy in the United States regarding its recreational and medicinal use is constantly evolving, cannabis remains one of the most used substances. THC has the most psychoactive effect of the cannabinoids and plays a role in the potency. Recent findings suggest high THC content in recreational cannabis, in conjunction with prolonged frequent use and dysregulation of the endocannabinoid system plus other factors, contribute to the development of cannabinoid hyperemesis syndrome (CHS).[52]

CHS represents a clinical syndrome of cyclical nausea, vomiting, and abdominal cramping in the setting of chronic cannabis use, typically relieved by taking a hot shower.[53] Patients often seek emergency medical treatment when hot showers no longer provide relief. Although the exact pathophysiology remains uncertain, two main theories exist: chronic overstimulation of the endocannabinoid receptors leading to derangements in intrinsic control of nausea and vomiting from central and peripheral sources and inactivation of the transient receptor potential vanilloid 1 nociceptor system in the peripheral nervous system.[53] CHS might respond to supportive care and usual anti-emetics. Some evidence supports capsaicin cream and haloperidol.[52,54] Cessation of cannabis use usually results in full recovery.[52]

There have been several case reports of cannabinoid-associated pancreatitis, the pathophysiology of which seems to be poorly understood.[55–57] Endocannabinoid receptors are found on the islet of Langerhans cells in the pancreas, and agonism at those receptors from exogenous cannabinoids likely plays a role.[58]

COCAINE

Cocaine is extracted from *Erythroxylum coca*. Cocaine is highly addictive, and its users may experience euphoria, sympathomimetic effects, CNS stimulation, vasoconstriction, vasospasm, and thrombus formation. Abdominal pain overall seems to be relatively infrequent in the cocaine user and are most likely to be associated with vascular pathologies.

Intestinal ischemia secondary to cocaine use has been reported and can cause significant morbidity and mortality.[59,60] The exact pathogenesis of organ ischemia remains unclear, but the theoretic etiology is profound mesenteric vasoconstriction.[61] Deep ulcerations of the gut may also occur and result in significant gastrointestinal bleeding or perforation of a viscus.[61–63] Patients with viscus perforation typically present with sudden, sharp epigastric pain with occasional referred shoulder pain.[61] Less commonly, they present with nausea, vomiting, and diarrhea with vague abdominal discomfort. The pathogenesis has yet to be fully elucidated, but consideration is given to focal ischemia secondary to vasoconstriction.[64]

Hepatic necrosis resembling ischemic hepatitis may occur following cocaine use, although there is some speculation that toxic cocaine metabolites may directly contribute.[15,65] Patients may have evidence of hepatotoxicity following an acute overdose.[65] Reported cases include elevated liver transaminases, elevated lactate dehydrogenase, elevated INR, and potential progression to fulminant liver failure or death.[66–68] One case noted an associated thrombotic microangiopathy with cocaine-induced acute hepatitis.[68] Hepatic injury in a patient with a cocaine use history may be multifactorial including damage from common hepatotoxins such as acetaminophen, other substances of abuse, adulterants or concomitant development of viral hepatitis from injection drug use.[69,70]

Lastly, there are rare reports of cocaine-associated pancreatitis, although this is quite difficult to isolate. Pathophysiology is multifactorial. It is thought to be the result of vasoconstriction and thrombotic microangiopathy of the mesenteric vessels, presynaptic nerve endings with elevated amounts of norepinephrine or indirectly related to levamisole-adulterated cocaine leading to an associated vasculitis.[59,70,71] Patients may present with typical signs and symptoms of pancreatitis as previously denoted. Other etiologies of pancreatitis must be considered before making this diagnosis.

Appropriate control, benzodiazepines as needed, avoidance of beta-adrenergic antagonists, and surgical consultation should be highly considered in the aforementioned cases.

KETAMINE AND PHENCYCLIDINE

Chronic ketamine use has been associated with abdominal and pelvic pain, usually from a urologic cause and potentially manifesting as hemorrhagic cystitis.[72] Less commonly, gastrointestinal pathology such as cholestasis, biliary dyskinesia, and upper abdominal pain with symptoms of gastritis has been described.[72] Elevated transaminases may signify hepatobiliary dysfunction from ketamine.[73] Abstinence from ketamine use should lead to recovery.

Phencyclidine is a similar xenobiotic with mostly CNS manifestations in acute toxicity and is not known to be directly toxic to the gastrointestinal tract. However, hyperthermia, hypovolemia and hypoxia may occur and lead to ischemic hepatitis.[74] Treatment is largely supportive.

RECOMMENDATIONS

As with any patient with abdominal pain, the approach to diagnosis and management needs to remain broad until a thorough history, physical examination, and testing can exclude emergent conditions, narrow the focus and management to the determined diagnosis. Patients with substance use disorders need to be approached in such a way that the physician or provider can establish good rapport, and the patient does not feel the stigma that can arise with a substance use disorder. Consultation and or referral to an addiction specialist to aid in management of the substance use disorder will be helpful to address and try to prevent any recurrence of disease.

SUMMARY

Patients with substance use disorders present commonly to the ED for illnesses related to their substance use. Often these illnesses include abdominal and gastrointestinal complaints. Alcohol use disorder and patients with OUD can have a wide range of diagnoses leading to ED visits such as gastritis, hepatitis, motility dysfunction, and pancreatitis. These patients should have complete history, physical examination, laboratory, and imaging studies to evaluate gastrointestinal emergencies based on their chief complaints. Treatment should focus on symptom relief or control and management of the underlying etiology of their illness. Patients should be assessed for motivation to seek aid for their substance use disorders as both a treatment and prevention of future episodes of illness.

CLINICS CARE POINTS

- Alcoholic liver disease exists on a spectrum with minimal gastrointestinal symptoms to near-death from upper gastrointestinal hemorrhage
- In the absence of other risk factors or obvious causes, use of cocaine and amphetamine derivatives may be implicated in hepatic ischemia, bowel ischemia, and viscus perforation
- Cannabinoids and cocaine have rarely been associated with pancreatitis
- With significant hepatotoxicity or hepatic failure of unclear etiology, consideration should be given to hepatitis or chronic use of hepatotoxins such as ethanol, MDMA, cocaine, amphetamines, or acetaminophen-containing compounds
- Hyperalgesia resulting from chronic opioid use can be associated with narcotic bowel syndrome and opioid withdrawal
- Aggressive bowel regimens for patients on chronic opioids should be considered
- Symptomatic and supportive care are the mainstays of treatment in opioid withdrawal which often manifest with abdominal complaints, although consideration should be given to medication-assisted treatment in the right candidate

DISCLOSURE

The authors have nothing to disclose. There are no funding sources to disclose.

REFERENCES

1. Rui P, Kang K. National Hospital Ambulatory Medical Care Survey: 2017 emergency department summary tables. National Center for Health Statistics. Available at: https://www.cdc.gov/nchs/data/nhamcs/web_tables/2017_ed_web_tables-508.pdf. Accessed January 28, 2021.
2. Mahajan G. Role of Urine Drug Testing in the Current Opioid Epidemic. Anesth Analg 2017;125(6):2094–104.
3. Bode C, Bode JC. Alcohol's role in gastrointestinal tract disorders. Alcohol Health Res World 1997;21(1):76–83.
4. Miller SC, Fiellin DA, Rosenthal RN. Gastrointestinal disorders related to alcohol or other drug use. In: The ASAM principles of addiction medicine. 6th edition. Lippincott Williams and Wilkins; 2018.
5. Meseeha M, Attia M. Esophageal Varices. In: StatPearls. 2020. Available at: https://www.ncbi.nlm.nih.gov/books/NBK448078/. Accessed January 31, 2021.
6. Turner AR, Turner SD. Boerhaave Syndrome. In: StatPearls. 2020. Available at: https://www.ncbi.nlm.nih.gov/books/NBK430808/. Accessed January 31, 2021.
7. Zhang L, Eslick GD, Xia HHX, et al. Relationship between Alcohol Consumption and Active *Helicobacter pylori* Infection. Alcohol Alcohol 2010;45(1):89–94.
8. Rosenstock S, Jorgensen T, Bonnevie O, et al. Risk factors for peptic ulcer disease: a population based prospective cohort study comprising 2416 Danish Adults. Gut 2003;52:186–93.
9. Mohy-ud-din N, Morrissey S. Pancreatitis. In: StatPearls. 2020. Available at: https://www.ncbi.nlm.nih.gov/books/NBK538337/. Accessed January 31, 2021.
10. Banks PA, Bollen TL, Dervenis C, et al. Classification of acute pancreatitis - 2012: Revision of the Atlanta classification and definitions by international consensus. Gut 2013;62(1):102–11.
11. Singh VK, Yadav D, Garg PK. Diagnosis and Management of Chronic Pancreatitis: A Review. JAMA 2019;322(24):2422–34.
12. Samokhvalov AV, Rehm J, Roerecke M. Alcohol Consumption as a Risk Factor for Acute and Chronic Pancreatitis: A Systematic Review and a Series of Meta-analyses. EBioMedicine 2015;2(12):1996–2002.
13. Barry K. Chronic Pancreatitis: Diagnosis and Treatment. Am Fam Physician 2018; 97(6):385–93.
14. Patel R, Mueller M. Alcoholic Liver Disease. In: StatPearls. 2020. Available at: https://www.ncbi.nlm.nih.gov/books/NBK546632/. Accessed February 1, 2021.
15. Haber PS, Freyer CH. Liver disorders related to alcohol and other drug use. In: Miller SC, Fiellin DA, Rosenthal RN, et al, editors. The ASAM principles of addiction medicine. Wolters-Kluwer: 6th edition. Lippincott Williams and Wilkins; 2018.
16. Rocco A, Compare D, Angrisani D, et al. Alcoholic disease: liver and beyond. World J Gastroenterol 2014;20(40):14652–9.
17. Al-Rabadi L, Al Marj C, et al. Renal and metabolic disorders related to alcohol and other drug use. In: Miller SC, Fiellin DA, Rosenthal RN, et al, editors. The ASAM principles of addiction medicine. Wolters-Kluwer: 6th edition. Lippincott Williams and Wilkins; 2018.
18. Medici V, Halsted CH. Folate, alcohol, and liver disease. Mol Nutr Food Res 2013; 57(4):596–606.

19. Yip L. Ethanol. In: Nelson L, Howland MA, Lewin NA, et al. McGraw-Hill Education. Goldfrank's Toxicologic Emergencies. 11th edition. 2019. p. 1143 - 1156.
20. Howard RD, Bokhari SRA. Alcoholic Ketoacidosis. Jan 2020 In: StatPearls. Available at: https://www.ncbi.nlm.nih.gov/books/NBK430922/. Accessed February 1, 2021.
21. de Menezes RF, Bergmann A, Thuler LC. Alcohol consumption and risk of cancer: a systematic literature review. Asian Pac J Cancer Prev 2013;14(9):4965–72.
22. Peck J, Replete N, Melquist S, et al. Adolescent With Acute Liver Failure in the Setting of Ethanol, Cocaine, and Ecstasy Ingestion Treated With a Molecular Adsorbent Recirculating System. Cureus 2020;12(8):e9699.
23. Nelson L, Olsen D. Opioids. In: Nelson L, Howland MA, Lewin NA, et al. McGraw-Hill Education. Goldfrank's Toxicologic Emergencies. 11th edition; 2019.p. 519 - 537.
24. Kan D, Zweben J, Stine S, et al. Pharmacological and psychosocial treatment for opioid use disorder. In: Miller SC, Fiellin DA, Rosenthal RN, et al, editors. The ASAM principles of addiction medicine. Wolters-Kluwer: 6th Edition. Lippincott Williams and Wilkins; 2018.
25. Kong EL, Burns B. Narcotic Bowel Syndrome. In: StatPearls. 2020. Available at: https://www.ncbi.nlm.nih.gov/books/NBK493207/. Accessed January 28 2021.
26. Grunkemeier DM, Cassara JE, Dalton CB, et al. The narcotic bowel syndrome: clinical features, pathophysiology, and management. Clin Gastroenterol Hepatol 2007;5(10):1126–39.
27. Haber PS, Elsayed M, Espinoza D, et al. Constipation and other common symptoms reported by women and men in methadone and buprenorphine maintenance treatment. Drug Alcohol Depend 2017;181:132–9.
28. Webster LR, Camilleri M, Finn A. Opioid-induced constipation: rationale for the role of norbuprenorphine in buprenorphine-treated individuals. Subst Abuse Rehabil 2016;7:81–6.
29. Sizar O, Genova R, Gupta M. Opioid Induced Constipation. In: StatPearls. 2020. Available at: https://www.ncbi.nlm.nih.gov/books/NBK493184/. Accessed January 28, 2021.
30. Ratuapli SK, Crowell MD, DiBaise JK, et al. Opioid-Induced Esophageal Dysfunction (OIED) in Patients on Chronic Opioids. Am J Gastroenterol 2015;110(7): 979–84.
31. Camilleri M, Lembo A, Katzka D. Opioids in Gastroenterology: Treating Adverse Effects and Creating Therapeutic Benefits. Clin Gastroenterol Hepatol 2017;15: 1338–49.
32. Ho V, Stewart M, Boyd P. Cholestatic hepatitis as a possible new side-effect of oxycodone: a case report. J Med Case Rep 2008;2:140.
33. LiverTox. Clinical and Research Information on Drug-Induced Liver Injury [Internet]. Bethesda (MD): National Institute of Diabetes and Digestive and Kidney Diseases. Available at: https://www.ncbi.nlm.nih.gov/books/NBK547955/. Accessed February 1, 2021.
34. Liang TJ, Ward JW. Hepatitis C in Injection-Drug Users - A Hidden Danger of the Opioid Epidemic. N Engl J Med 2018;378:1169–71.
35. Trickey A, Fraser H, Lim A, et al. The Contribution of Injection Drug Use to Hepatitis C Virus Transmission Globally, Regionally, and at Country Level: A Modelling Study. Lancet Gastroenterol Hepatol 2019;4(6):435–44.
36. Candy B, Jones L, Vickerstaff V, et al. Mu-opioid antagonists for opioid-induced bowel dysfunction in people with cancer and people receiving palliative care. Cochrane Database Syst Rev 2018;6(6):CD006332.

37. Leppert W. Oxycodone/naloxone in the management of patients with pain and opioid-induced bowel dysfunction. Curr Drug Targets 2014;15(1):124–35.

38. Yuan C, Foss JF, O'Connor M, et al. Methylnaltrexone for Reversal of Constipation Due to Chronic Methadone Use: A Randomized Controlled Trial. JAMA 2000; 283(3):367–72.

39. Leppert W. Emerging therapies for patients with symptoms of opioid-induced bowel dysfunction. Drug Des Devel Ther 2015;9:2215–31.

40. Garnock-Jones KP. Naloxegol: a review of its use in patients with opioid-induced constipation. Drugs 2015;75(4):419–25.

41. Lugoboni F, Mirijello A, Zamboni L, et al. High prevalence of constipation and reduced quality of life in opioid-dependent patients treated with opioid substitution treatments. Expert Opin Pharmacother 2016;17(16):2135–41.

42. Shah M, Huecker MR. Opioid Withdrawal. In: StatPearls [Internet]. 2020. Available at: https://www.ncbi.nlm.nih.gov/books/NBK526012/. Accessed January 29, 2021.

43. Vasan S, Olango GJ. Amphetamine Toxicity. In: StatPearls. 2020. Available at: https://www.ncbi.nlm.nih.gov/books/NBK470276/. Accessed February 1, 2021.

44. Steinkellner T, Freissmuth M, Sitte HH, et al. The ugly side of amphetamines: short- and long-term toxicity of 3,4-methylenedioxymethamphetamine (MDMA, 'Ecstasy'), methamphetamine and D-amphetamine. Biol Chem 2011;392(1–2): 103–15.

45. Green PA, Battersby C, Heath RM, et al. A fatal case of amphetamine induced ischaemic colitis. Ann R Coll Surg Engl 2017;99(7):e200–1.

46. Zou XM, Huang HM, Yang LM, et al. Methamphetamine consumption and life-threatening abdominal complications. Medicine 2018;97(18):e0647.

47. Ciupilan E, Gapp M, Stelzl R, et al. Amphetamine-induced small bowel ischemia - A case report. Radiol Case Rep 2020;15(11):2183–7.

48. Gavriilidis G, Kyriakoudi A, Tiniakos D, et al. Bath Salts" intoxication with multiorgan failure and left-sided ischemic colitis: a case report. Hippokratia 2015;19(4): 363–5.

49. Panikkath R, Panikkath D. Amphetamine-related ischemic colitis causing gastrointestinal bleeding. Proc Bayl Univ Med Cen 2016;29(3):325–6.

50. Johnson TD, Berenson MM. Methamphetamine-induced ischemic colitis. J Clin Gastroenterol 1991;13(6):687–9.

51. Moore PW, Donovan JW. ACMT- Methamphetamine. Available at: https://www. acmt.net/Methamphetamine_FAQ.html. Accessed January 28, 2021.

52. Sorensen CJ, DeSanto K, Borgelt L, et al. Cannabinoid Hyperemesis Syndrome: Diagnosis, Pathophysiology, and Treatment-a Systematic Review. J Med Toxicol 2017;13(1):71–87.

53. Chu F, Cascella M. Cannabinoid Hyperemesis Syndrome. In: StatPearls. 2020. Available at: https://www.ncbi.nlm.nih.gov/books/NBK549915/. Accessed January 28 2021.

54. Moon AM, Buckley SA, Mark NM. Successful Treatment of Cannabinoid Hyperemesis Syndrome with Topical Capsaicin. ACG Case Rep J 2018;5:e3.

55. Grant P, Gandhi P. A case of cannabis-induced pancreatitis. JOP 2004;5(1):41–3.

56. Wargo KA, Geveden BN, McConnell VJ. Cannabinoid-induced pancreatitis: a case series. JOP 2007;8(5):579–83.

57. Fatma H, Mouna B, Leila M, et al. Cannabis: a rare cause of acute pancreatitis. Clin Res Hepatol Gastroenterol 2013;37(1):e24–5.

58. Akkucuk MH, Erbayrak M. A Rare and Unexpected Side-Effect of Cannabis Use: Abdominal Pain due to Acute Pancreatitis. Case Rep Emerg Med 2015;2015: 463836.
59. Carlin N, Nguyen N, DePasquale J. Multiple Gastrointestinal Complications of Crack Cocaine Abuse. Case Rep Med 2014;2014:512939.
60. Muñiz AE, Evans T. Acute gastrointestinal manifestations associated with use of crack. Am J Emerg Med 2001;19:61–3.
61. Chander B, Aslanian HR. Gastric perforations associated with the use of crack cocaine. Gastroenterol Hepatol (N Y) 2010;6(11):733–5.
62. Wattoo MA, Osundeko O. Cocaine-induced intestinal ischemia. West J Med 1999;170(1):47–9.
63. Gibbons TE, Sayed K, Fuchs GJ. Massive pan-gastrointestinal bleeding following cocaine use. World J Pediatr 2009;5(2):149–51.
64. Nalbandian H, Sheth N, Dietrich R, et al. Intestinal ischemia caused by cocaine ingestion: report of two cases. Surgery 1985;97(3):374–6.
65. LiverTox: Clinical and Research Information on Drug-Induced Liver Injury [Internet]. Bethesda (MD): National Institute of Diabetes and Digestive and Kidney Diseases; 2012. Cocaine. Available at: https://www.ncbi.nlm.nih.gov/books/NBK548454/. Accessed February 1, 2021.
66. Kanel GC, Cassidy W, Shuster L, et al. Cocaine-induced liver cell injury: comparison of morphological features in man and in experimental models. Hepatology 1990;11:646–51.
67. Balaguer F, Fernández J, Lozano M, et al. Cocaine-induced acute hepatitis and thrombotic microangiopathy. JAMA 2005;293(7):797–8.
68. Adedinsewo D, Ajao O, Okpobrisi O, et al. Acute cocaine-induced hepatotoxicity with features of shock liver. Case Rep Clin Pathol 2015;2(4).
69. Edlin BR, Carden MR. Injection drug users: the overlooked core of the hepatitis C epidemic. Clin Infect Dis 2006;42(5):673–6.
70. Ogunbameru A, Jandali M, Issa A, et al. Acute pancreatitis as initial presentation of cocaine-induced vasculitis: a case report. JOP 2015;16(2):192–4.
71. Umar M, Noor E, Ali U, et al. Cocaine-Induced Acute Pancreatitis: A Rare Etiology. Cureus 2020;12(7):e9029.
72. Pappachan JM, Raj B, Thomas S, et al. Multiorgan dysfunction related to chronic ketamine abuse. Proc (Bayl Univ Med Cent) 2014;27(3):223–5.
73. Olmedo R. Phencyclidine and ketamine. In: Nelson L, Howland MA, Lewin NA, et al. McGraw-Hill Education. Goldfrank's Toxicologic Emergencies, 11th edition. 2019.p.1210 - 1221.
74. LiverTox: Clinical and Research Information on Drug-Induced Liver Injury [Internet]. Bethesda (MD): National Institute of Diabetes and Digestive and Kidney Diseases; 2012. Phencyclidine. Available at: https://www.ncbi.nlm.nih.gov/books/NBK548654/. Accessed February 1, 2021.

Abdominal Pain Mimics

Neeraja Murali, DO, MPH[a],*, Sahar Morkos El Hayek, MD[b]

KEYWORDS

- Abdominal pain • Mimics • Differential diagnosis

KEY POINTS

- Abdominal pain is the most common reason for emergency department visits in the United States.
- Abdominal pain mimics are conditions that present with abdominal pain but are not caused by gastrointestinal abnormalities.
- Emergency physicians should keep abdominal pain mimics on the differential to avoid missing life-threatening diagnoses.

INTRODUCTION

Abdominal complaints comprise up to 10% of emergency department visits.[1] Abdominal pain can be the presenting symptom of potentially serious diagnoses that may not be caused by gastrointestinal pathology, but rather by mimics with extra-gastrointestinal origin (**Box 1**). In this article, we discuss some of these alternative causes of abdominal pain.

Although some of these pathologies cause abdominal pain because of their location within the abdominopelvic cavity, others have varying mechanisms. Some have shared visceral innervation, whereas others present with gastrointestinal symptoms such as nausea, vomiting, and diarrhea. Still, others involve cellular pathways resulting in irregularities to the gastrointestinal (GI) tract. When assessing a patient with abdominal complaints, it is important to have a broad differential diagnosis to identify these nongastrointestinal conditions.

CAN'T-MISS DIAGNOSES: ACUTE LIFE THREATS
Acute Coronary Syndrome

Coronary artery disease is consistently the leading cause of death in the United States.[2] Acute coronary syndrome (ACS) manifests as chest pain in 40% to 75% of cases, but can have atypical presentations including nausea, vomiting, and abdominal pain, leading to misdiagnosis and undertreatment.[3,4] Symptoms may vary based on

[a] Department of Emergency Medicine, University of Maryland School of Medicine, 110 S Paca Street, 6th Floor, Suite 200, Baltimore, MD 21201, USA; [b] Washington University in Saint Louis, 660 S Euclid Avenue CB 8072, St Louis, MO 63110, USA
* Corresponding author.
E-mail address: nmurali@som.umaryland.edu

Emerg Med Clin N Am 39 (2021) 839–850
https://doi.org/10.1016/j.emc.2021.07.003
0733-8627/21/© 2021 Elsevier Inc. All rights reserved.

emed.theclinics.com

Box 1
Selected abdominal pain mimics by category

Cardiovascular/Pulmonary
  Acute coronary syndrome
  Aortic dissection
  Congestive heart failure
  Pneumonia
  Pulmonary embolism
  Ruptured abdominal aortic aneurysm
Environmental
  Black widow spider bite
  Envenomation
  Heat stroke
  Mushroom toxicity
Functional
  Cyclic vomiting syndrome
  Irritable bowel syndrome
Hematologic
  Neutropenic enterocolitis
  Porphyria
  Sickle cell crises
  Spontaneous splenic rupture
Immunologic/Vasculitic
  Angioedema
  Food allergies
  Henoch-Schonlein purpura
  Polyarteritis nodosa
  Systemic lupus erythematosus

Genitourinary
  Ectopic pregnancy
  Ovarian torsion
  Pyelonephritis
  Testicular torsion
  Tubo-ovarian abscess
  Uremia
Infectious
  COVID-19
  Herpes zoster
  Lemierre's syndrome
  Lyme disease
  Pneumonia
Metabolic
  Adrenal crisis
  Alcoholic ketoacidosis
  Diabetic ketoacidosis
  Hypercalcemia
  Hyperglycemic emergencies
  Pheochromocytoma
  Thyrotoxicosis
Neurologic
  Abdominal epilepsy
  Abdominal migraine
Toxic
  Heavy metal poisoning
  Substance intoxication/withdrawal

---

patient demographics, and certain patients, particularly the elderly, women, and diabetics can present with atypical symptoms. These atypical symptoms are likely due to the shared visceral sensory innervation between the heart and GI tract, making the location of pain less sensitive in the diagnosis of ACS. Emergency physicians should have a low threshold to rule out ACS in high-risk patients presenting with nonspecific abdominal pain. Work-up for ACS includes an electrocardiogram and cardiac enzymes. If cardiac etiology is ruled out, further investigation into other etiologies is warranted.

Aortic Emergencies

The major life-threatening acute aortic syndromes encountered by emergency physicians are aortic dissection (AD) and ruptured abdominal aortic aneurysm (AAA). Although uncommon, these entities carry a high mortality rate due in part to their variable presentations and absence of diagnostic laboratory testing.[5] Survival depends on rapid diagnosis and treatment.[6] ADs typically present with tearing chest and back pain, but can present with isolated abdominal pain, especially in type B dissections. Ruptured or symptomatic AAAs present primarily with acute, severe abdominal pain associated with hemoperitoneum, usually causing hemodynamic instability. Risk factors for aortic pathology include male gender and age more than 63 years.[7] History of hypertension, smoking, and known connective tissue disorders are also predisposing factors. Evaluation often begins with cardiac work-up, and a chest x-ray may show a widened mediastinum in type A AD. Bedside ultrasound should be considered to evaluate for flap in AD or for aortic enlargement with or without hemoperitoneum in AAA, particularly in unstable patients. This modality is 99% sensitive and 98% specific in identifying AAA greater than 3 cm in diameter.[8] In stable patients, contrast-enhanced computed tomography angiography (CTA) is the imaging modality of choice to diagnose and guide management of ADs and aneurysms.[9]

Pulmonary Embolism

Venous thromboembolism (VTE) accounts for 100,000 to 180,000 deaths annually in the United States.[10] Mortality approaches 30% if undiagnosed compared to a 2.5% to 10% when appropriately diagnosed and treated.[11,12] Patients with pulmonary embolism (PE) can present with a variety of symptoms, including pleuritic chest pain, dyspnea on exertion, hemoptysis, or even circulatory collapse.[13] However, nearly 6.7% of patients with PE seek medical attention for vague gastrointestinal complaints.[12] The mechanism by which PE causes abdominal pain is unclear, but may be related to hepatic congestion from right heart strain and distention of the liver capsule or diaphragmatic irritation from pulmonary infarction.[14–16]

Multiple clinical decision tools can be implemented to risk-stratify patients for PE. Known malignancy, use of exogenous estrogens, prolonged immobilization, and known hypercoagulable state raise the concern for VTE. In patients with atypical presentations where there is a high concern for PE, clinical decision rules should not be applied. Notably, thrombosis is a relatively common complication of COVID-19 infection, with a disproportionate incidence of PE, believed to be caused by pulmonary microthrombi.[17,18] Instead chest CTA should be pursued to avoid missing this life-threatening diagnosis.

Ectopic Pregnancy

Ectopic pregnancy (EP) is the implantation of a fertilized egg outside the endometrium, most commonly in the fallopian tube. It occurs in 1% to 2% of all pregnancies and can cause hemorrhagic shock and maternal death.[19] The classic symptoms are abdominal/pelvic pain, vaginal bleeding, or amenorrhea, but presentation is often nonspecific.[19–21] Hypotension with vaginal bleeding in a woman of reproductive age is highly concerning for ruptured EP. Risk factors include age over 35 years, smoking, prior history of EP, tubal luminal injury from prior infections, and pregnancy with assisted reproduction.[19,22] A beta-human chorionic gonadotropin (beta-hCG) above the discriminatory zone without ultrasound evidence of intrauterine pregnancy should prompt further evaluation for EP. Management in hemodynamically stable patients consists of medical treatment with methotrexate. Surgical intervention is indicated in hemodynamically unstable patients or those with contraindications to methotrexate.

Ovarian Torsion

Ovarian torsion (OT) represents 2.7% of all gynecologic emergencies, with an incidence of 4.9 per 100,000 before the age of 20 years.[23] This diagnosis is often missed because of its nonspecific presentation of acute onset abdominal pain associated with nausea and vomiting.[24] Physicians should maintain a high index of suspicion for OT, as late or missed diagnosis can result in ovarian loss and reduced fertility. Gynecologic and surgical history is of utmost importance, as OT remains a clinical diagnosis confirmed only with laparoscopy. Physical examination is usually nonspecific but can elicit an enlarged abdominal mass. Transvaginal ultrasound with doppler is the initial test of choice to evaluate for OT, and the most consistent finding is an enlarged edematous ovary with a "string of pearls" sign.[25,26] Ultrasound may also show a lack of blood flow to the affected ovary (**Fig. 1**).[27] Other findings include a "whirlpool sign," large ovarian cysts, and pelvic free fluid.[25–27] Computed tomography (CT) and MRI can be used when abdominal pathology is still on the differential. However, laparoscopy remains the diagnostic gold standard for OT.[28] Laparoscopy for detorsion and oophoropexy is the treatment of choice to salvage the ovary in premenopausal women.[22–28]

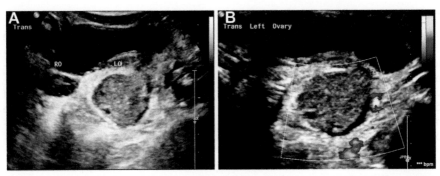

Fig. 1. Ovarian torsion in a prepubescent female. (*A*) Left ovary (LO) and right ovary (RO) on gray-scale transverse US. Note the significant difference in size, with the left ovary measuring 18.8 mL while the right measures 3.9 mL. The left ovary also has peripheral follicles and hyperechoic fat, suggesting mesenteric fat stranding. (*B*) Image of the left ovary with no intraovarian flow as seen on power Doppler. (From Ngo AV, Otjen JP, Parisi MT, et al. Pediatric ovarian torsion: a pictorial review. Pediatr Radiol 2015;45(12):1845-55; with permission.)

Hyperglycemic Emergencies

Diabetic ketoacidosis (DKA) and hyperglycemic hyperosmolar state (HHS) are 2 conditions that are life-threatening if not recognized and managed promptly. DKA accounts for 50% of deaths in diabetics under the age of 21 years; however, overall mortality rates for DKA remain less than 1%.[29] HHS, on the other hand, has an inpatient mortality rate of up to 16%.[29] DKA and HHS present with abdominal pain, nausea, and vomiting, which often resolve with the correction of the underlying metabolic derangements. Pain does not correlate with the severity of hyperglycemia, but may be related to acidosis or precipitating factors such as toxic ingestions, pancreatitis, infection, or dehydration.[30] Management of both conditions involves aggressive hydration, insulin, electrolyte replacement, and addressing the underlying cause.[31]

Adrenal Crisis

Acute adrenal crisis has an incidence of up to 10 per 100 patient-years and a mortality rate approaching 0.5/100 patient-years. It is more likely to occur in patients with primary adrenal insufficiency than in patients with secondary adrenal insufficiency. Acute adrenal crisis is often incited by (commonly viral gastrointestinal illness) or abrupt cessation of chronic steroids. Early symptoms include fever, nausea, vomiting, and lower abdominal pain. Physical examination may reveal signs of Cushing's disease and even findings of an acute abdomen. If left untreated, patients will progress to hypotension and altered mental status, consistent with shock, and ultimately to cardiovascular collapse.[32] Laboratory findings include hyponatremia, hypoglycemia, and hyperkalemia, sometimes reflected on EKG. Adrenocorticotropic hormone and cortisol levels can confirm diagnosis, though the treating clinician should not wait for these results. Management includes directed therapy for shock, expeditious glucocorticoids, and supportive care.[33]

SHOULDN'T-MISS DIAGNOSES: REQUIRE URGENT AND TIMELY INTERVENTION
Congestive Heart Failure Exacerbation

Heart failure is a common presentation to the emergency department. Acute exacerbation of heart failure is the gradual or rapid decompensation of cardiac function, resulting from either fluid overload or maldistribution. Common presenting symptoms include dyspnea, orthopnea, and edema. A subset of patients present with nonspecific abdominal pain, especially children and adolescents with dilated cardiomyopathy.[34] These symptoms, which include right upper quadrant (RUQ) pain, nausea, and vomiting, are thought to be due to congestive hepatopathy from fluid overload and can mimic biliary colic, cholecystitis, and hepatitis. Fluid overload causing splanchnic congestion leads to bowel wall edema, ileus, and possibly bowel ischemia. Severe heart failure exacerbation resulting in cardiogenic shock can present with abdominal pain due to nonocclusive mesenteric ischemia. A proposed mechanism is the combination of preferential shunting of blood from mesenteric circulation to cardiac and cerebral circulation and the concomitant mesenteric vasospasm.[35] If serious abdominal pathologies are ruled out and symptoms are attributed to heart failure, the typical treatment includes acute diuresis and cardiac optimization.

Pneumonia

Pneumonia is a common respiratory infection, and its diagnosis is among the mainstays of emergency medicine. Although classic symptoms include cough, chest pain, and fevers, it is important to remember that at extremes of age, the presenting features may vary. In these groups, symptoms are more likely to include headache, nausea, and abdominal pain.[36] The diagnosis of pneumonia can be made based on symptoms, imaging, and clinical examination findings, and treatment should be targeted toward the most likely organisms in the particular patient. Pneumonia is a common cause of sepsis and early and aggressive treatment should be considered to minimize the risk of deterioration.[36]

COVID-19

The SARS-CoV-2 virus has been associated with a wide array of symptoms which cause the syndrome known as COVID-19. Among the manifestations of COVID-19 are diarrhea, nausea, vomiting, and abdominal pain, which can be present in up to 50% of patients evaluated for COVID-19. Symptoms are hypothesized to be due to binding of viral particles to angiotensin-converting enzyme-2 (ACE-2) receptors within the GI tract.[37] Notably, GI symptoms may present later in disease course than respiratory symptoms. Patients with COVID-19 may exhibit elevated liver function tests (LFTs) and bilirubin, with higher elevations in more severe illness.[38] ACE-2 receptors are also expressed in pancreatic islet cells, and a pancreatitis-like presentation may thus be seen.[39] Management strategies for COVID-19 are rapidly evolving as knowledge about the syndrome improves.

Pelvic Inflammatory Disease

Pelvic inflammatory disease (PID) is the inflammation of the upper female reproductive tract induced by an infection ascending from the vagina or cervix.[40] *Chlamydia trachomatis* and *Neisseria gonorrhea* are the most commonly implicated organisms. Patients present with pelvic or abdominal pain of varying severity, vaginal discharge, dyspareunia, and postcoital bleeding.[40] In severe cases, patients can present with fever and RUQ pain due to liver capsule inflammation and adhesions, known as Fitz-Hugh-Curtis syndrome. Timely clinical diagnosis of PID is crucial, as prolonged infection and inflammation can lead to infertility and increase the risk of EP. PID is a clinical diagnosis based on pelvic examination findings of cervical motion tenderness, adnexal tenderness, and mucopurulent cervical discharge. Transvaginal ultrasound can be used to confirm the diagnosis.[41] Laparoscopic diagnosis remains the gold standard but is not routinely performed. Most patients can be treated as outpatients, except during pregnancy, presence of tubo-ovarian abscess, or severe illness with inability to tolerate oral antibiotics. A single dose of intramuscular ceftriaxone followed by oral doxycycline for 2 weeks is the current recommended outpatient treatment, while parenteral treatment consists of cefotetan or cefoxitin with doxycycline.[40,42,43]

Sickle Cell Crises

Patients with sickle cell disease (SCD) often present to the emergency department due to complications of their disease. SCD is caused by morphologically abnormal erythrocytes. Abdominal pain is attributed to microvascular occlusion causing infarcts of the visceral and mesenteric structures within the abdomen. Most common among these is vaso-occlusive pain crisis. Abdominal pain is one of the most frequent symptoms associated with these pain crises and often mimics an acute abdomen.[44] The pain of vaso-occlusive crisis can progress to hepatic, splenic, and renal infarcts, with laboratory and imaging studies reflecting these pathologies. Once intra-abdominal pathology has been excluded, it is reasonable to treat the patient for vaso-occlusive crisis. Analgesia is paramount, and intravenous fluids should be considered only if the patient shows signs of hypovolemia.[45]

Multiple RUQ pathologies are associated with SCD. The hemolysis in SCD leads to the formation of pigmented gallstones, which in turn increase the risk of symptomatic cholelithiasis and acute cholecystitis. These sickled red blood cells can also occlude hepatic sinuses and ducts. The resultant acute intrahepatic cholestasis can lead to derangements in hepatic and renal function or coagulation abnormalities. A severe consequence of SCD is acute sickle hepatic crisis, which affects up to 10% of those admitted for abdominal pain crises and often mimics acute cholecystitis.[45] In patients with SCD and RUQ, the clinician should have a low threshold to obtain hepatic function tests, coagulation panels, and appropriate imaging, especially with associated physical examination findings.

Splenic sequestration (and eventual infarct) is commonly seen in SCD, particularly in children. Sequestration is defined as splenomegaly with a hemoglobin drop of ≥ 2 g/dL from baseline. It can rapidly progress and lead to shock. Repeated episodes may require splenectomy. Oftentimes, patients undergo splenic autoinfarction and atrophy before the age of 5 years.[46] Asplenia leaves patients with SCD at increased risk of infection by encapsulated organisms. In patients who present for evaluation with a history of SCD, other pathologies including acute chest and aplastic crisis should also be considered before assuming vaso-occlusive crisis.[47]

Thyrotoxicosis

Thyrotoxicosis is another uncommon diagnosis that can present with abdominal pain. The annual incidence of 30 cases per 100,000. If left untreated, it can lead to thyroid storm, which has a mortality rate of up to 50%.[48] Thyrotoxicosis is associated with gastroparesis, resulting in nausea, vomiting, and abdominal pain. Other symptoms can be consistent with a hypermetabolic state with increased sympathetic drive.[49] The causes of vomiting in thyrotoxicosis are unclear, but may be related to the action of thyroid hormones on GI motility.[48] A common presenting sign is tachycardia, and laboratory derangements may include abnormal LFTs in addition to thyroid studies consistent with hyperthyroidism.[50] Excess thyroid hormone is thought to have direct and secondary effects on the liver, leading to hepatocellular damage. Treatment includes beta-blockade and antithyroid agents such as propylthiouracil and methimazole, with relatively rapid return to normal function.[48]

Uremia

Uremia describes the spectrum of conditions and illnesses associated with kidney failure that are not otherwise explained by the disease state. It is the accumulation of metabolic waste products that are typically cleared by normal kidneys. The treatment of uremia is primarily via dialysis, and 5-year survival for dialysis patients is under 35%.[51] Early signs and symptoms of uremia are vague, and may include fatigue, anorexia, nausea, and anemia, among many other symptoms.[51] As the disease progresses, multiple organ systems may become involved. The initiation of dialysis is often heralded by worsening gastrointestinal symptoms, and symptoms such as dysgeusia and distaste for specific foods may suggest the need to initiate dialysis. Patients may also manifest signs and symptoms consistent with malnutrition. Although dialysis can temper metabolic derangements and improve survival, the long-term prognosis is poor without successful renal transplantation.[52]

WILL MISS IF NOT CONSIDERED: UNCOMMON PRESENTATIONS AND RARE DIAGNOSES

Acute Intermittent Porphyria

Porphyrias are a group of syndromes which arise from a defect in heme synthesis. The most common and severe of these syndromes is acute intermittent porphyria (AIP). It is an autosomal dominant condition with incomplete penetrance; as such, symptomatic disease is only seen in 1 to 2/100,000.[53] Triggers include drugs, infection, alcohol, steroids, and fasting. In AIP, neurovisceral crises due to failures in the heme synthetic pathway present as severe, colicky, epigastric pain with vomiting and constipation. Patients may progress to having psychiatric symptoms as well as peripheral and autonomic neuropathies mimicking Guillain-Barre Syndrome. The diagnosis can be confirmed with the measurement of urine porphobilinogen, aminolevulinic acid, and porphyrins from a sample during an acute attack. This sample should be shielded from light, as these molecules are photosensitive. Patients may present with hyponatremia, hypomagnesemia, slight leukocytosis, and elevated aminotransferases.[54] If AIP is suspected, consider the patient's urine color; with this condition, colorless or yellow urine will turn dark red or purple within hours if exposed to light.[55] AIP flares are managed conservatively with sugar or carbohydrate boluses and definitive treatment is via heme transfusions.

Lead Toxicity

Lead toxicity is a rare cause of abdominal pain; however, missing the diagnosis can lead to severe morbidity and mortality. Abdominal pain due to lead toxicity is usually subacute, intermittent, located in the upper quadrants, and associated with constipation.[56] Lead toxicity can also present with anemia, hearing loss, neurotoxicity, and death. Blood lead level (BLL) >5 μg/dL is considered elevated.[57] As lead exposure is commonly occupational and environmental, treatment starts with limiting exposures. BLL over 70 μg/dL requires chelating agents such as dimercaprol, DMSA, and D-penicillamine.

Henoch–Schönlein Purpura

Henoch–Schönlein Purpura (HSP) is a systemic, small vessel vasculitis caused by the deposition of IgA in vessel walls of the skin, gastrointestinal tract, joints, and kidneys. It is the most common vasculitis in children, with an incidence of 10 to 20 cases per 100,000 children/year.[58] It is a self-limited condition that lasts an average of 4 weeks.[59] The classic HSP tetrad is cutaneous palpable purpura, joint pain, gastrointestinal complaints, and renal involvement. GI presentations range from colicky abdominal pain to intussusception, bowel ischemia, and perforation.[60] Prognosis and long-term sequelae depend on the extent of renal involvement, ranging from isolated microscopic hematuria, to nephritis complicated by nephrotic syndrome and end-stage renal disease. Treatment for HSP without renal involvement is symptomatic, including fluids and pain control. HSP nephritis is commonly treated with corticosteroids or other immunomodulators.

Hereditary Angioedema

Hereditary angioedema (HAE) is a rare autosomal dominant disorder, caused by C1-inhibitor deficiency. This deficiency contributes to a pathway that ultimately leads to vascular permeability and extravasation of plasma into interstitial tissue, causing non-pitting edema of the subcutaneous and submucosal tissue of the gastrointestinal and respiratory tracts and skin.[61,62] HAE attacks are precipitated by trauma, stress, and hormonal dysregulation. These attacks can appear as skin swelling, upper airway edema, and obstruction, and most commonly abdominal attacks, which occur in 80% of patients with HAE due to intestinal wall edema.[63] Symptoms include severe pain, nausea, vomiting, and distention. Attacks last up to 8 days and often resolve spontaneously.[64]

Work-up for HAE includes measuring plasma C4 and C-1 inhibitor levels. CT scans of the abdomen during an attack will show bowel wall edema and ascites but are nondiagnostic.[65]

In addition to symptomatic management, the first-line treatment for acute attacks includes C1-inhibitor replacement, a bradykinin B2-receptor antagonist, or a kallikrein inhibitor. Fresh frozen plasma is second-line therapy.[66]

Shingles

In herpes zoster, pain often precedes the presence of rash. Although the pain typically involves a single dermatome, it can also involve 2 or 3 consecutive dermatomes. It does not typically cross the midline.[67] The vesicles that develop will usually crust over in 7 to 10 days. Outbreaks can be managed with antivirals such as acyclovir or valacyclovir. Patients will often present with postherpetic neuralgia, which follows the same dermatomal distribution but persists for at least 90 days after acute infection. Symptoms can be managed with topical agents, oral gabapentin, or pregabalin. Vaccination should be considered if clinically appropriate.[68]

Abdominal Migraine

Abdominal migraine is a diagnosis of exclusion. It is typically seen in childhood and is characterized by episodic central abdominal pain associated symptoms usually associated with migraines: nausea, vomiting, pallor, and photophobia. However, headaches are not usually present. Adults are not likely to have a first-time diagnosis of abdominal migraine unless there is a strong family history.[69] It is often associated with other cyclic conditions such as cyclic vomiting syndrome. Acute symptoms resolve in more than 80% of patients with rest in a dark, quiet room.[70] Some limited evidence shows that pizotifen may be of benefit if medication is needed.[70]

SUMMARY

Non-gastrointestinal causes of abdominal pain should be considered before assigning a diagnosis of nonspecific abdominal pain. This article is by no means exhaustive and there are many diagnoses to be considered. Although some of these can be made in the emergency department, some will require appropriate outpatient follow-up. A high index of suspicion is needed when evaluating patients with abdominal pain.

CLINICS CARE POINTS

- Thorough history and physical examination are mainstays of diagnosis and should help guide any interventions and testing.
- Serial abdominal examinations can help with both diagnosis and treatment.
- If a diagnosis is in doubt, strong return precautions and expeditious follow-up are essential.
- Patients, particularly those at extremes of age may present with atypical presentations of life-threatening conditions.
- Having a broad differential across multiple organ systems can help prevent anchoring bias in the evaluation of patients.

DISCLOSURES

Dr Murali received an honorarium for a brief discussion on appendicitis on the podcast "Emergency Medicine: Reviews and Perspectives," published February 2021. No other disclosures.

REFERENCES

1. Rui P, Kang K. National hospital ambulatory medical care survey: 2017 emergency department summary tables. National Center for Health Statistics. Available at: https://www.cdc.gov/nchs/data/nhamcs/web_tables/2017_ed_web_tables-508.pdf. Accessed June 29, 2021.
2. Products - Data Briefs - Number 254-August 2016. Cdc.gov. 2021. Available at: https://www.cdc.gov/nchs/products/databriefs/db254.htm. Accessed January 29, 2021.
3. Chang A, Fischman D, Hollander J. Evaluation of chest pain and acute coronary syndromes. Cardiol Clin 2018;36(1):1–12.
4. Brieger D, Eagle K, Goodman S, et al. Acute coronary syndromes without chest pain, an underdiagnosed and undertreated high-risk group. Chest 2004;126(2):461–9.
5. Upchurch G, Nienaber C, Fattori R, et al. Acute aortic dissection presenting with primarily abdominal pain: a rare manifestation of a deadly disease. Ann Vasc Surg 2005;19(3):367–73.
6. Linett L. Dissecting abdominal aortic aneurysm in a young man: an uncommon presentation of abdominal pain. Am J Emerg Med 2005;23(3):383–5.
7. Lo C, Chen C, Hsueh C, et al. Aortic dissection mimics acute abdomen in an older patient. Int J Gerontol 2012;6(2):140–3.
8. Rubano E, Mehta N, Caputo W, et al. Systematic review: emergency department bedside ultrasonography for diagnosing suspected abdominal aortic aneurysm. Acad Emerg Med 2013;20(2):128–38.
9. Baliyan V, Parakh A, Prabhakar A, et al. Acute aortic syndromes and aortic emergencies. Cardiovasc Diagn Ther 2018;8(S1):S82–96.
10. Goldhaber S. Venous thromboembolism: epidemiology and magnitude of the problem. Best Pract Res Clin Haematol 2012;25(3):235–42.
11. Calder K, Herbert M, Henderson S. The mortality of untreated pulmonary embolism in emergency department patients. Ann Emerg Med 2005;45(3):302–10.

12. Derr C, Gantner J, Keffeler J. Pulmonary embolism: an abdominal pain masquerader. J Emerg Trauma Shock 2013;6(4):280.
13. Stein P, Beemath A, Matta F, et al. Clinical characteristics of patients with acute pulmonary embolism: data from PIOPED II. Am J Med 2007;120(10):871–9.
14. von Pohle W. Pulmonary embolism presenting as acute abdominal pain. Respiration 1996;63(5):318–20.
15. Herbert A. Pathogenesis of pleurisy, pleural fibrosis, and mesothelial proliferation. Thorax 1986;41(3):176–89.
16. Dalen J, Haffajee C, Alpert J, et al. Pulmonary embolism, pulmonary hemorrhage and pulmonary infarction. N Engl J Med 1977;296(25):1431–5.
17. Scudiero F, Silverio A, Di Maio M, et al. Pulmonary embolism in COVID-19 patients: prevalence, predictors and clinical outcome. Thromb Res 2021;198:34–9.
18. Vlachou M, Drebes A, Candilio L, et al. Pulmonary thrombosis in Covid-19: before, during and after hospital admission. J Thromb Thrombolysis 2021; 51(4):978–84.
19. Panelli D, Phillips C, Brady P. Incidence, diagnosis and management of tubal and nontubal ectopic pregnancies: a review. Fertil Res Pract 2015;1:15.
20. Robertson J, Long B, Koyfman A. Emergency medicine myths: ectopic pregnancy evaluation, risk factors, and presentation. J Emerg Med 2017;53(6): 819–28.
21. Lawani O, Anozie E. Ectopic pregnancy: a life-threatening gynecological emergency. Int J Womens Health 2013;515.
22. Jurkovic D, Wilkinson H. Diagnosis and management of ectopic pregnancy. BMJ 2011;342(1):d3397.
23. Guthrie B, Adler M, Powell E. Incidence and trends of pediatric ovarian torsion hospitalizations in the United States, 2000-2006. Pediatrics 2010;125(3):532–8.
24. Houry D, Abbott J. Ovarian torsion: a fifteen-year review. Ann Emerg Med 2001; 38(2):156–9.
25. Ashwal E, Krissi H, Hiersch L, et al. Presentation, diagnosis, and treatment of ovarian torsion in premenarchal girls. J Pediatr Adolesc Gynecol 2015;28(6): 526–9.
26. Damigos E, Johns J, Ross J. An update on the diagnosis and management of ovarian torsion. The Obstet Gynaecol 2012;14(4):229–36.
27. Ngo AV, Otjen JP, Parsis MT, et al. Pediatric ovarian torsion: a pictorial review. Pediatr Radiol 2015;45(12):1845–55.
28. Sasaki K, Miller C. Adnexal torsion: review of the literature. J Minim Invasive Gynecol 2014;21(2):196–202.
29. Fayfman M, Pasquel F, Umpierrez G. Management of hyperglycemic crises. Med Clin North Am 2017;101(3):587–606.
30. Umpierrez G, Freire A. Abdominal pain in patients with hyperglycemic crises. J Crit Care 2002;17(1):63–7.
31. Elzouki A, Eledrisi M. Management of diabetic ketoacidosis in adults: a narrative review. Saudi J Med Med Sci 2020;8(3):165.
32. Rathbun KM, Nguyen M, Singhal M. Addisonian Crisis. In: StatPearls. Treasure Island (FL): StatPearls Publishing; 2020.
33. Fares A, Santos R. Conduct protocol in emergency: acute adrenal insufficiency. Rev Assoc Méd Bras 2016;62(8):728–34.
34. Hollander SA, Addonizio LJ, Chin C, et al. Abdominal complaints as a common first presentation of heart failure in adolescents with dilated cardiomyopathy. Am J Emerg Med 2013;31(4):684–6.

35. Al-Diery H, Phillips A, Evennett N, et al. The pathogenesis of nonocclusive mesenteric ischemia: implications for research and clinical practice. J Intensive Care Med 2019;34(10):771–81.
36. Grief SN, Loza JK. Guidelines for the evaluation and treatment of pneumonia. Prim Care 2018;45(3):485–503.
37. Wong SH, Lui RN, Sung JJ. Covid-19 and the digestive system. J Gastroenterol Hepatol 2020;35(5):744–8.
38. Patel KP, Patel PA, Vunnam RR, et al. Gastrointestinal, hepatobiliary, and pancreatic manifestations of COVID-19. J Clin Virol 2020;128:104386.
39. Saeed U, Sellevoll HB, Young VS, et al. Covid-19 may present with acute abdominal pain. Br J Surg 2020;107(7):e186–7.
40. Brunham RC, Gottlieb SL, Paavonen J. Pelvic inflammatory disease. N Engl J Med 2015;372(21):2039–48.
41. Romosan G, Valentin L. The sensitivity and specificity of transvaginal ultrasound with regard to acute pelvic inflammatory disease: a review of the literature. Arch Gynecol Obstet 2014;289(4):705–14.
42. Savaris RF, Fuhrich DG, Maissiat J, et al. Antibiotic therapy for pelvic inflammatory disease. Cochrane Database Syst Rev 2020;8:CD010285.
43. Pelvic Inflammatory Disease (PID) - 2015 STD treatment guidelines. 2015 sexually transmitted diseases treatment guidelines. 2015. Available at: https://www.cdc.gov/std/tg2015/pid.htm. Accessed May 31, 2021.
44. Ahmed S, Shahid R, Russo L. Unusual causes of abdominal pain: sickle cell anemia. Best Pract Res Clin Gastroenterol 2005;19(2):297–310.
45. Simon E, Long B, Koyfman A. Emergency medicine management of sickle cell disease complications: an evidence-based update. J Emerg Med 2016;51(4):370–81.
46. Bender MA. Sickle cell disease. In: Adam MP, Ardinger HH, Pagon RA, et al, editors. GeneReviews®. Seattle (WA): University of Washington; 2003.
47. Borhade MB, Kondamudi NP. Sickle cell crisis. In: StatPearls. Treasure Island (FL): StatPearls Publishing; 2020.
48. Hoogendorn E, Cools B. Hyperthyroidism as a cause of persistent vomiting. Neth J Med 2021;62(8):293–6.
49. Gharahbaghian L, Brosnan D, Fox J, et al. New onset thyrotoxicosis presenting as vomiting, abdominal pain and transaminitis in the emergency department. West J Emerg Med 2007;8(3):97–100.
50. Rotman-Pikielny P, Borodin O, Zissin R, et al. Newly diagnosed thyrotoxicosis in hospitalized patients: clinical characteristics. QJM 2008;101(11):871–4.
51. Meyer T, Hostetter T. Uremia. N Engl J Med 2007;357(13):1316–25.
52. Almeras C, Argilés À. The general picture of uremia. Semin Dial 2009;22(4):329–33.
53. Herrick AL, McColl KE. Acute intermittent porphyria. Best Pract Res Clin Gastroenterol 2005;19(2):235–49.
54. Gonzalez-Mosquera LF, Sonthalia S. Acute intermittent porphyria. In: StatPearls. Treasure Island (FL): StatPearls Publishing; 2020.
55. Yuan T, Li YH, Wang X, et al. Acute intermittent porphyria: a diagnostic challenge for endocrinologist. Chin Med J (Engl) 2015;128(14):1980–1.
56. Moriarity RS, Harris JT, Cox RD. Lead toxicity as an etiology for abdominal pain in the emergency department. J Emerg Med 2014;46(2):e35–8.
57. Shabani M, Hadeiy SK, Parhizgar P, et al. Lead poisoning; a neglected potential diagnosis in abdominal pain. BMC Gastroenterol 2020;20(1):134.

58. Gardner-Medwin JM, Dolezalova P, Cummins C, et al. Incidence of Henoch-Schönlein purpura, Kawasaki disease, and rare vasculitides in children of different ethnic origins. Lancet 2002;360(9341):1197–202.
59. Saulsbury FT. Henoch-Schönlein purpura. Curr Opin Rheumatol 2010;22(5): 598–602.
60. Hetland LE, Susrud KS, Lindahl KH, et al. Henoch-Schönlein purpura: a literature review. Acta Derm Venereol 2017;97(10):1160–6.
61. Zuraw BL. Clinical practice. Hereditary angioedema. N Engl J Med 2008;359(10): 1027–36.
62. Kaplan AP, Joseph K. The bradykinin-forming cascade and its role in hereditary angioedema. Ann Allergy Asthma Immunol 2010;104(3):193–204.
63. Jalaj S, Scolapio JS. Gastrointestinal manifestations, diagnosis, and management of hereditary angioedema. J Clin Gastroenterol 2013;47(10):817–23.
64. Roche O, Blanch A, Caballero T, et al. Hereditary angioedema due to C1 inhibitor deficiency: patient registry and approach to the prevalence in Spain. Ann Allergy Asthma Immunol 2005;94(4):498–503.
65. Locascio EJ, Mahler SA, Arnold TC. Intestinal angioedema misdiagnosed as recurrent episodes of gastroenteritis. West J Emerg Med 2010;11(4):391–4.
66. Zuraw BL, Busse PJ, White M, et al. Nanofiltered C1 inhibitor concentrate for treatment of hereditary angioedema. N Engl J Med 2010;363(6):513–22.
67. Dayan RR, Peleg R. Herpes zoster - typical and atypical presentations. Postgrad Med 2017;129(6):567–71.
68. Saguil A, Kane S, Mercado M, et al. Herpes zoster and postherpetic neuralgia: prevention and management. Am Fam Physician 2017;96(10):656–63.
69. Roberts JE, deShazo RD. Abdominal migraine, another cause of abdominal pain in adults. Am J Med 2012;125(11):1135–9.
70. Angus-Leppan H, Saatci D, Sutcliffe A, et al. Abdominal migraine. BMJ 2018;360: k179.

Diagnoses of Exclusion in the Workup of Abdominal Complaints

Joseph Wesley Watkins IV, MD*, Zachary Bert Lewis, MD

KEYWORDS

- Gastroparesis • Cyclic vomiting syndrome • Functional gallbladder
- Abdominal migraine • Gastroenteritis

KEY POINTS

- Familiarity with diagnoses of exclusion is useful in the evaluation for abdominal pain in the emergency department.
- Judiciously applied, these diagnoses of exclusion provide insight into patterns and pathology in patients with often repeated nondiagnostic visits to the emergency department.
- Understanding when to institute specific therapies and referrals for diseases such as gastroparesis, cyclic vomiting, or abdominal migraines can improve quality of life and even mortality.

INTRODUCTION

Abdominal pain is a common complaint in the emergency department (ED), comprising 8.8% of all visits.[1] Despite advances in medicine and imaging, 20% to 30% of patients still leave the department without a definitive diagnosis, and in fact, the most common discharge diagnosis for nontraumatic abdominal pain in the United States is nonspecific abdominal pain,[2] which can be distressing for patients who are seeking answers and unsatisfying for providers who would like to provide guidance. A working knowledge of diagnoses of exclusion (DOE) can help guide therapeutics and specialty referrals that may ultimately provide answers and relief. Overapplication of DOE can also present challenges, as providers can become victims of anchoring bias or of a need to provide an unfounded answer due to discomfort with the unknown. This concern is supported by the findings that in patients with a nonspecific diagnosis in the ED, 9% of those patients will be admitted or represented to the ED.[2]

Although not exhaustive, the following are the several commonly encountered abdominal DOE that often present acutely.

Drs J.W. Watkins and Z.B. Lewis have no commercial or financial conflicts of interest to disclose.
University of Arkansas for Medical Sciences, 4301 West Markham Street Slot 584, Little Rock, AR 72205, USA
* Corresponding author.
E-mail address: Jwwatkins@uams.edu

https://doi.org/10.1016/j.emc.2021.07.010
0733-8627/21/© 2021 Elsevier Inc. All rights reserved.
emed.theclinics.com

ACUTE GASTROENTERITIS

Acute gastroenteritis (AGE) is a common presentation to clinics and EDs in the United States, with an estimated 179 million cases, 500,000 hospitalizations, and 5000 deaths per year. Although it is assumed that AGE is an infectious process, only about 20% of patients who present for care have a causative organism identified.[3] The diagnosis of AGE is one of the exclusions in the ED.

AGE is generally defined as ≥1 episode of vomiting and ≥3 episodes of diarrhea over a 24-h period and may be associated with abdominal pain (76%) and fevers (32%).[4,5] It is primarily a disease of children, and its prevalence decreases by decade, with patients less than 5 year old more than three times as likely to be diagnosed with AGE than those greater than 65 year old.[5] Local outbreaks or travel to countries with inadequate sanitation can be suggestive of AGE.[6]

AGE is considered an inflammatory response to an infectious process within the gastrointestinal tract, resulting in nausea, vomiting and diarrhea among other symptoms.[3] Rarely is a causative organism identified, a factor of both limitations of testing and AGE's self-limiting nature. In those with an identified organism, a vast majority of AGE is viral in origin, with norovirus alone representing up to 50% of all cases.[7] Bacterial infections (**Table 1**) can exhibit more concerning features. Parasitic infections (**Box 1**) can cause more persistent symptoms (>14 days).[6]

The initial evaluation in the ED should focus on assessment of the patient's hydration status. Signs of systemic illness (fevers, sepsis), bloody or mucoid diarrhea, or significant abdominal pain suggest a more severe pathology and require a more thorough diagnostic evaluation. The 2017 IDSA guidelines suggest this evaluation include stool testing for pathogens, though this may not be feasible in the ED.[6] Hemolytic Uremic Syndrome (HUS) is a rare but dangerous complication of infectious diarrhea related mostly (90%) to Shiga-toxin producing E. coli (STEC). HUS evaluation should include hemoglobin, platelet count and assessment of renal function. Notably, bloody diarrhea often precedes laboratory abnormalities by several days, stressing the importance of outpatient follow up.[8] Infections, particularly with Yersinia, can present with focal abdominal pain and mesenteric adenitis often mimicking appendicitis.[9]

Persistent symptoms (14–29 days), immune suppression or patients with HIV/AIDS without a clear causative agent may benefit from gastroenterology follow up for colonoscopy or more comprehensive stool testing.[6]

AGE is generally self-limiting, and diarrhea (bloody or non-bloody) for <7 days in an immunocompetent patient does not require empiric antibiotics. Empiric treatment with a fluroquinolone or azithromycin should be reserved for infants less than 3 months, ill immunocompromised patients with a fever and abdominal pain, and international travelers with a fever.[6]

Ondansetron is encouraged in the acute phase of AGE.[6] It has been shown to decrease vomiting, need for intravenous (IV) rehydration and immediate hospitalization in these patients, though it may contribute to worsening diarrhea and did not decrease hospitalization at 72 hours.[10,11] Antimotility agents are discouraged in children and in patients with bloody diarrhea or fever. Adults with watery diarrhea without fever (ie, low risk of developing toxic megacolon) may receive loperamide.[6]

CYCLIC VOMITING SYNDROME

Cyclic vomiting syndrome (CVS) is an incompletely understood disease process that likely represents multiple causative entities grouped under a single umbrella.[12] The Rome IV criteria defined CVS as short (less than 1 week), recurrent (at least twice in past 6 months), sporadic (episodes at least 1 week apart) and stereotypical

Table 1
Common pathogens in bloody/mucoid diarrhea and their associations[6]

Pathogen	Campylobacter	Yersinia	Shigella	Salmonella	Shiga Toxin–Producing E coli (STEC)
Association	Undercooked poultry	Undercooked pork, right lower quadrant pain	Feco-oral transmission	Exposure to reptiles, foodborne outbreaks	Hemolytic Uremic Syndrome (HUS)

episodes of vomiting.[13] Currently encompassed by this broad definition is the emerging subgroup of cannabinoid hyperemesis syndrome (CHS), which has been increasing in frequency in parallel to looser regulations on the use of cannabis in the United States.[14]

The true prevalence of CVS is unknown, but a small, survey-based study suggested it affects up to 2% of the US population, with a slight male predominance.[12,15] There is often significant delay in diagnosis for these patients, with an average of 5 ED visits prior to diagnosis.[16] An association between CVS and personal or family history of migraine headaches has been established, which informs some of the empiric treatments currently recommended.[12]

These patients present with intermittent, stereotypical episodes of vomiting and oral intolerance. Some patients have specific triggers that may provoke attacks. These can include psychiatric stress, menses, sleep deprivation and even "pleasant excitement". There are often prodromal phases during which patients can abort an attack. Prodromal symptoms can include sweating, food aversion, abdominal pain, insomnia, and irritability.[17] Once patients progress to the vomiting/retching phase of their attack, it can be difficult to treat and often precipitates visits to the ED.

Consensus definition for CVS was first offered in 2006, and exploration into its pathophysiology is still in its infancy.[18] Given its strong association with migraine headaches, and shared features with seizure disorders (cyclical symptom onset with prodromal phase and inter-episodic quiescent phase), experts have focused on CVS as a possible neurogenic disorder, as opposed to gastrointestinal.[12] This is further supported by reported benefits of antiepileptics and antimigraine medications.[19] Specific genetic mutations have been associated with CVS in children, though in adults this association is less clear.[20] Autonomic dysfunction has a known association with CVS, suggesting a role for the sympathetic nervous system.[16]

Box 1
Parasites associated with persistent diarrheal illness[6]

Cryptosporidium

Giardia

Trichinella

Cyclospora

Cystoisospora

Microsporidia

The endocannabinoid system may also have a role in CVS. Small studies have demonstrated an increase in endocannabinoid lipids during acute episodes of CVS.[21] In CHS, the further suggestion is that increased potency of cannabinoid products, coupled with chronic use may downregulate cannabinoid receptors and lower the threshold for an episode in vulnerable patients.[12]

Perhaps the easiest way to sort through the litany of putative causes of CVS attacks is to consider a cyclic vomiting "threshold", not unlike a seizure threshold, above which an attack is provoked. The combination of above factors (genetics, stressors, autonomic dysfunction, endocannabinoids) all likely impact an individual's cyclic vomiting threshold and should be considered and treated in concert to prevent morbidity.[19]

Diagnosis of CVS on an index visit to the ED would be unreasonable. Consideration of advanced imaging for intra-abdominal pathology (small bowel obstruction, volvulus, perforated peptic ulcer, etc) would be prudent. Likewise, laboratory values assessing for hydration status, electrolyte depletion, biliary obstruction or pancreatitis can be helpful. Although usage patterns of cannabinoids needed to provoke CHS are not well established, a detailed history of use should be obtained.

After multiple stereotypic presentations in patients with previously unrevealing workups, one should consider the diagnosis of CVS. In addition to an in-depth history to establish patterns, triggers and associated symptoms, CVS patients will generally have an outpatient structural assessment with an esophageal gastroduodenoscopy and a functional assessment of gastric emptying.[17]

Recommendation for treatment regimens of CVS is based on poor quality studies and anecdotal evidence. Survey studies have shown that up to 89% of patients believed that CVS was not recognized by the ED, despite an existing diagnosis, reinforcing a need for knowledge translation.[16] The Cyclic Vomiting Syndrome Association has published consensus management guidelines for CVS that hope to standardize the approach to these patients (**Table 2**).[22] If patients present early after symptom onset (within 60 minutes), abortive therapies including intranasal or intramuscular sumatriptan as well as aprepitant or ondansetron can be effective. Recommendations for treatment in the ED consist of a stepwise approach, starting with crystalloid infusion, ondansetron, diphenhydramine, metoclopramide, and IV fosaprepitant (NK1 antagonist, if available). If symptoms persist, moving to sedatives such as lorazepam is appropriate. Avoid opioids when possible. Butyrophenones (haloperidol, droperidol) have limited data, suggesting improved outcomes in the treatment of CHS. A small, 33-patient study comparing haloperidol (at 0.1 mg/kg and 0.05 mg/kg dose) with ondansetron (8 mg) found improved treatment success and decreased time to discharge in those treated with haloperidol.[23] Similarly, droperidol was associated with decreased length of stay in a retrospective study of ED patients with CHS.[24]

Table 2
Therapeutics in cyclic vomiting syndrome[22]

Preventative	Abortive	Emergency Treatment
Tricyclic Antidepressants	Sumatriptan	Ondansetron
Topiramate	Ondansetron	Metoclopramide
Zonisamide	Aprepitant	Diphenhydramine
Levetiracetam	-	Fosaprepitant
Aprepitant	-	Lorazepam

ABDOMINAL MIGRAINE

Abdominal migraine (AM) is a rare disorder and an infrequently recognized cause of abdominal pain and gastrointestinal symptoms. Although AM was initially researched and reported in the context of migraine headache, AM can present independently of headache. Prevalence is estimated at 1% to 4% in children aged 3 to 15 years with a mean age of onset of 7 years.[25,26] Prevalence tends to decrease with age although adult cases have been reported.[27]

The patients with AM present with recurrent episodes of intense, acute abdominal pain and a combination of nausea, vomiting, anorexia, and pallor.[28] Diagnostic criteria have been set forth by the Rome group (**Box 2**).[29] The abdominal pain in AM can be variable; it may be described as midline, periumbilical, poorly localized, or a more generalized soreness or dull pain. In the absence of a known history of AM, the physical examination may raise concern for early visceral abdominal pain or mild, generalized peritonitis. If focality is present, further workup should be strongly considered. AM and CVS share some similar symptoms, although important differences can be noted including demographics for certain younger age groups and specific social history considerations. Both disorders have asymptomatic periods.[30]

The pathophysiology of AM remains ill-defined. Despite ambiguous origins, AM has shown a genetic and psychosocial component that cannot be ignored.[31] AM is classified as a functional gastrointestinal disorder. The visceral hyperalgesia hypothesis applied to such conditions suggests that these disorders are related to alteration of the brain-gut axis and abnormal secretion of excitatory neurotransmitters due to increased sensitizations of sensory neurons, altered inhibitory control, and an impaired stress response.[32] Briefly, it suggests an exaggerated gastrointestinal response to both physiologic and psychosocial stress. Another hypothesis parallels the more well-known and studied migrainous processes with the suggestion that an imbalance of neurotransmitters and their metabolism leads to symptoms.[33]

Treatment of the patient's symptoms before consideration of imaging is reasonable. If imaging can be deferred based on recurrent, episodic nature of presentation or relatively benign examination, the ED workup can be limited to general screening based on demographics and risk factors. Urine analysis is essential in the screening process, especially in younger children and urine pregnancy test in appropriate patients.

Box 2
Rome III criteria for abdominal migraines[29]

1. At least 2 sudden onset episodes of intense, acute periumbilical pain within the last 6 months lasting at least 1 hour and should be most distressing symptom

2. Symptom-free periods of usual health lasting weeks to months

3. The pain is severe enough to limit normal activities

4. Pattern of symptoms and progression develops for individual patient

5. The pain is associated with 2 or more of the following:
   a. Anorexia
   b. Nausea
   c. Vomiting
   d. Headache
   e. Photophobia
   f. Pallor

6. No other alternative process can adequately explain the subject's symptoms

Gastrointestinal fluid losses will likely not be as prominent as those seen in CVS, but significant dehydration or electrolyte abnormalities will require treatment. Alarming symptoms have been suggested to alert of more insidious pathology and include fever, bloody vomitus or stool, and localization of pain.[32]

Because patients are free from symptoms between episodes, outpatient workup can be difficult. The ED physician should focus on recognizing the alarming symptoms that suggest an alternative pathology, and referring for any necessary further evaluation. AM can have variable combinations and degrees of symptoms, but once the AM diagnostic criteria have been satisfied, this diagnosis can be strongly considered and treated.

In general, the treatment of AM focuses on acute management of episodes and prophylaxis. Acute management from the ED should start with oral analgesics and antiemetics. Standard analgesics and antiemetics can be used, but the same serotonergic and dopaminergic medications that treat migrainous processes, such as prochlorperazine, may have more success in treating symptoms.[34] Prophylactic medications include serotonin agonists, beta-blockers, ergots, and antiepileptics, but these medications should be provided through a primary care physician or specialist. Patients also benefit from an understanding of their diagnosis, possible psychosocial triggers, and avoidance strategies.[35]

GASTROPARESIS

Gastroparesis is a challenging and incompletely understood entity that represents a significant burden to EDs.[36] Unlike other DOE discussed in this chapter, gastroparesis does in fact have objective criteria for diagnosis: objective evidence of delayed gastric emptying without underlying mechanical obstruction. By virtue of the inability to obtain these measurements in the ED, it can often be a diagnosis of exclusion in the ED.

Using the aforementioned strict definition, gastroparesis afflicts approximately 24 per 100,000 people in the United States. However, multiple studies have suggested that the actual prevalence of gastroparesis is as high as 2% of the population, with up to 90% of patients going undiagnosed.[37,38] There has been a trend toward increasing ED utilization in these patients, with a doubling of patients with an ED discharge diagnosis of gastroparesis from 2006 to 2013.[37]

Classically, GP is associated with diabetes mellitus, but recent data suggest that 39% to 50% of diagnosed GP is classified as idiopathic.[39] Other frequent causes of gastroparesis are drug-induced, postsurgical, postviral, or radiation associated.[40]

Advances in the understanding of gastroparesis pathophysiology over the past decade support a complex interplay between extrinsic and intrinsic innervation defects, diminished nitric oxide synthase, smooth muscle dysfunction, and fibrosis.[41] More recently, data have suggested the predominant role of an injury to the enteric nervous system, resulting in loss or dysfunction of the interstitial cells of Cajal, which are responsible for regulating smooth muscle contractility, leading to antral and small bowel dysmotility.[42]

The cardinal symptoms of gastroparesis are nausea, vomiting, early satiety, postprandial fullness, upper abdominal pain, and weight loss.[43] Nausea is the most predominant reported symptom of gastroparesis, with abdominal pain as the predominant symptom in up to 21% of patients.[44] Up to 50% of patients report that their symptoms began acutely.[45]

Functionally, acute gastroparesis behaves as other gastric outlet obstructions, with intractable emesis or retching, often combined with epigastric pain. Episodes of acute GP may be infrequent or may be cyclical.[46] Although unlike other types of recurrent functional abdominal pain (cyclic vomiting, cannabinoid hyperemesis) patients with gastroparesis generally have a more consistent course, with daily chronic complaints escalating to ED visits.[40]

A preexisting diagnosis of gastroparesis may make workup and management relatively simple. Given the prevalence of undiagnosed gastroparesis described earlier, it is likely that patients will present undifferentiated, requiring more thorough workup.

The patients with gastroparesis will present with obstructive gastrointestinal symptoms, and advanced abdominal imaging is often warranted on the index visit to rule out mechanical pathology. On subsequent ED visits with similar symptomatology, radiologic imaging has limited utility.[42] Pancreatitis or biliary complaints can also present with similar symptomatology and should be considered.

Gastric emptying can be measured via several mechanisms, none of which are feasible in the ED. Most commonly, gastric emptying is measured with scintigraphy of a radiolabeled solid meal at 2 hours after ingestion.[47] In recurrent cases, referral to a gastroenterology specialist is encouraged.

Although long-term therapies for gastroparesis can include gastric electrical stimulation, botulinum toxin injections, and pyloromyotomy, the mainstay of treatment of acute episodes of gastroparesis remains prokinetics and antiemetics.[41] Early studies demonstrated the efficacy of D2 antagonists/5-HT4 agonists, such as metoclopramide, in symptom improvement, and these drugs remain the only Food and Drug Administration–approved medication for gastroparesis.[48] 5-HT3 antagonists (eg, ondansetron) are also routinely used for nausea and vomiting associated with gastroparesis.[42] Although evidence is weak and varied, macrolide antibiotics do affect gastric motility and are used clinically. Their effectiveness is limited by side effects (QT prolongation, diarrhea) and tachyphylaxis.[49]

Recent studies have suggested a promising role of Haloperidol as an effective adjunct for treatment of gastroparesis in the ED.[50,51] Volume resuscitation with balanced crystalloid, as well as electrolyte repletion, may also improve gastric motility and improve symptoms of gastroparesis.[52,53]

IRRITABLE BOWEL SYNDROME

Irritable bowel syndrome (IBS) prevalence has been estimated at 5% to 15% of the US population although as many as 75% of IBS cases are clinically undiagnosed, and these prevalence rates have been determined by functional gastrointestinal surveys.[54,55] IBS symptoms can be divided into 4 subtypes based on bowel habit and stool consistency: constipation, diarrhea, mixed, or undefined.

Patients describe abdominal cramping and pain associated with an increase either in constipation or in diarrhea. Diagnostic criteria focus on changes of stool consistency and frequency around the onset of abdominal pain. Abdominal pain is a hallmark feature of IBS, and its absence suggests an alternative pathology.[56] Bloating and abdominal distension are commonly reported and have been the focus of various research studies as possible measurable examination features without convincing results.[57] Symptoms and examination findings are generally milder than those seen in gastroenteritis and CVS, which may correlate with the large portion of patients who do not seek diagnosis or medical care. Symptom onset can be related certain foods or stressors. IBS is more common among woman and patients younger than 50 years.[58]

As a functional gastrointestinal disorder, IBS does not have a definitive test for diagnosis. Its pathophysiology is poorly defined but is suggested to be related to hypersensitivity or impaired digestion of certain foods, particularly fermentable oligosaccharides, disaccharides and monosaccharides, and polyols (FODMAPs). Postinfectious states following *Escherichia coli* or *Giardia lamblia* may increase the risk for IBS, and microbial overgrowth of the small intestine has been suggested as a target for treatment.[59,60] Patients have had improved symptoms and symptom-free periods with dietary changes and avoidance strategies, although various studies have noted a confounding placebo effect could be present.[61]

In patients with a known diagnosis of IBS, it is warranted to elicit specific concerns that led the patient into the ED for evaluation, as changes in their chronic condition should allow a more directed workup. The examination should again focus on volume status assessment and evaluation of the severity and focality of abdominal tenderness. Imaging should only be obtained if surgical pathology is suggested on examination of the abdomen. Patients without the previous diagnosis of IBS will have symptoms similar to inflammatory bowel disease (IBD), which may heighten concern for hidden pathology.

Because of the prevalence of IBS, outpatient workup can coincide with treatment of IBS or even be deferred until initial treatments are attempted. Consideration of family history for IBD and careful review of red flag symptoms will help avoid missing alternative pathologies. Inflammatory markers have been proposed to help assist in differentiating IBS from IBD during acute episodes.[62] High-sensitivity inflammatory markers are now being studied to potentially differentiate patients with IBS from healthy controls.[63] IBS with constipation (IBS-C) should be differentiated from constipation due to colonic or rectal dysfunction that require evaluation by manometry or transit testing, as botulism injection or neurostimulator implants may be curative and not initially considered in the treatment of IBS-C.[64]

Patients with diagnosis of IBS will likely have a strong relationship with their primary care or gastroenterologist. If they present to the ED in relation to IBS, there is often a change from their normal symptoms or an urgent issue related to communication breakdown (ie, medication refill). Treatment from the ED should be focused on symptom management, which can often be recommendations for further outpatient treatments with prescriptions provided as necessary. Trends suggest that consistent outpatient follow-up and treatment decrease ED visits and specialist referrals from the ED. Most treatments start with dietary changes focused on increased fiber and decreased use but not elimination of FODMAPs. The only interventions noted to have strong evidence for use are tricyclic antidepressants and linaclotide, a peptide active in the gut with inhibition of pain receptors and increased luminal chloride, bicarbonate, and water. Strongly recommended treatments with weak to moderate evidence include rifaximin antibiotic, lubiprostone laxative for IBS-C subtype, and loperamide antidiarrheal for IBS-D subtype.[65]

FUNCTIONAL GALLBLADDER DISORDER

Nausea and vomiting associated with right upper quadrant abdominal pain raises the concern for gallbladder and liver pathology. Functional gallbladder disorders (FGD) are known by many terms including gallbladder dyskinesia, gallbladder spasm, acalculous biliary disease, chronic acalculous cholecystitis, chronic acalculous, gallbladder dysfunction, or cystic duct syndrome. Symptoms associated with FGDs can usually be controlled, and the ED workup is uncomplicated.

The history, examination, and diagnostic features proposed by the Rome criteria may assist with diagnosis of functional gallbladder and sphincter of Oddi disorders.[66] The Rome criteria reference biliary pain, typically described as sudden onset right upper quadrant abdominal pain that can radiate to the epigastrium, back, or right shoulder blade with a postprandial pattern. Although often referred to as "colicky," biliary pain is usually persistent although slightly improved at about 30 minutes after onset. To meet criteria for FGD, this pain must recur at variable intervals but not daily, and it must be severe enough to affect the patient's daily activities or lead to ED treatment.[67]

As a diagnosis of exclusion, the ED workup including liver function tests, lipase, and the providers choice of imaging must be unremarkable. Point-of-care ultrasound, radiology-performed ultrasound, and computed tomography imaging can all be used to exclude acute biliary emergencies including acute cholecystitis and cholangitis. When gallstones and inflammatory changes of the gallbladder are absent, FGD may be considered.

Outpatient workup may be pursued by either a primary care physician or gastroenterologist. They will need to treat common upper gastrointestinal issues such as reflux and ulcers and may coincide with consideration of alternative causes including FGDs. Endoscopic evaluation of upper gastrointestinal tract mucosa and endoscopic ultrasound evaluation of the cystic duct and biliary tree for microlithiasis can ensure alternate pathologies are not overlooked. Gallbladder ejection fractions can be calculated with hepatobiliary iminodiacetic acid(HIDA) scintigraphy. Standardized protocols for when to perform HIDA scans and how to perform HIDA scans are essential to limiting false-positive/-negative results.[68] Ejection fractions of less than 40% suggest dysfunction although recent case reports suggest that some patients with abnormally high ejection factures of greater than 90% had similar symptoms.[69]

Once alternative pathology has been excluded and abnormal gallbladder function is noted on HIDA scan, cholecystectomy may be considered. Recent research has suggested that the decision to proceed with surgery should be based on the degree of ejection fraction decrease and the similarity of patient's pain episodes to expected biliary pain.[70] Elective cholecystectomies for biliary dyskinesia are increasing in both adult and pediatric populations within the United States.[71,72] Some patients treated for presumed FGD with cholecystectomy continued to have similar symptoms and return ED visits despite gallbladder removal[73]; this suggests that some patients may not benefit from surgery and that the overall management of these patients should be focused on symptomatic treatment unless there is suspicion of more unusual, overlooked pathologies such as undiagnosed sphincter of Oddi dysfunction, missed stones, or tumor.[74]

SUMMARY

Although diagnoses of exclusion often fall outside of the diagnostic purview of the emergency physician, a working understanding of these diagnoses is essential. Patients whose complaints cannot be definitively diagnosed in the ED are often left hopeless and frustrated. It can take multiple ED visits (up to 150!) before a patient receives a final diagnosis and appropriate treatment.[16] These patients are more likely to miss work, lose their jobs, have a poorer quality of life, and have a shorter life expectancy.[75] Better recognition and careful application of these diagnoses can lead to improved symptomatic treatment and appropriate referrals that may improve lives.

REFERENCES

1. Rui P, Kang K. National Hospital Ambulatory Medical Care Survey: 2017 emergency department summary tables. National Center for Health Statistics. Available at: https://www.cdc.gov/nchs/data/nhamcs/web_tables?2-17_ed_web_tables-508.pdf. Accessed June 29, 2021.

2. Cervellin G, Mora R, Ticinesi A, et al. Epidemiology and outcomes of acute abdominal pain in a large urban Emergency Department: retrospective analysis of 5,340 cases. Ann Transl Med 2016;4(19):362.

3. Scallan E, Griffin PM, Angulo FJ, et al. Foodborne illness acquired in the United States–unspecified agents. Emerg Infect Dis 2011;17:16–22.

4. Bresee JS, Marcus R, Venezia RA, et al, US Acute Gastroenteritis Etiology Study Team. The etiology of severe acute gastroenteritis among adults visiting emergency departments in the United States. J Infect Dis 2012;205(9):1374–81.

5. Jones TF, McMillian MB, Scallan E, et al. A population-based estimate of the substantial burden of diarrhoeal disease in the United States; FoodNet, 1996-2003. Epidemiol Infect 2007;135(2):293–301.

6. Shane AL, Mody RK, Crump JA, et al. 2017 Infectious diseases society of america clinical practice guidelines for the diagnosis and management of infectious diarrhea. Clin Infect Dis 2017;65(12):e45–80.

7. Patel MM, Hall AJ, Vinjé J, et al. Noroviruses: a comprehensive review. J Clin Virol 2009;44(1):1–8.

8. Tarr PI, Gordon CA, Chandler WL. Shiga-toxin-producing Escherichia coli and haemolytic uraemic syndrome. Lancet 2005;365(9464):1073–86.

9. Saebø A. The Yersinia enterocolitica infection in acute abdominal surgery. A clinical study with a 5-year follow-up period. Ann Surg 1983;198(6):760–5.

10. Fedorowicz Z, Jagannath VA, Carter B. Antiemetics for reducing vomiting related to acute gastroenteritis in children and adolescents. Cochrane Database Syst Rev 2011;2011(9):CD005506.

11. Ramsook C, Sahagun-Carreon I, Kozinetz CA, et al. A randomized clinical trial comparing oral ondansetron with placebo in children with vomiting from acute gastroenteritis. Ann Emerg Med 2002;39(4):397–403.

12. Hasler WL, Levinthal DJ, Tarbell SE, et al. Cyclic vomiting syndrome: Pathophysiology, comorbidities, and future research directions. Neurogastroenterol Motil 2019;31(Suppl 2):e13607.

13. Stanghellini V, Chan FK, Hasler WL, et al. Gastroduodenal disorders. Gastroenterology 2016;150(6):1380–92.

14. Bhandari S, Jha P, Lisdahl KM, et al. Recent trends in cyclic vomiting syndrome-associated hospitalisations with liberalisation of cannabis use in the state of Colorado. Intern Med J 2019;49(5):649–55.

15. Aziz I, Palsson OS, Whitehead WE, et al. Epidemiology, clinical characteristics, and associations for Rome IV functional nausea and vomiting disorders in adults. Clin Gastroenterol Hepatol 2019;17:878–86.

16. Venkatesan T, Tarbell S, Adams K, et al. A survey of emergency department use in patients with cyclic vomiting syndrome. BMC Emerg Med 2010;10:4.

17. Fleisher DR, Gornowicz B, Adams K, et al. Cyclic Vomiting Syndrome in 41 adults: the illness, the patients, and prob- lems of management. BMC Med 2005;3:20.

18. Tack J, Talley NJ, Camilleri M, et al. Functional gastroduodenal disorders. Gastroenterology 2006;130(5):1466–79.

19. Levinthal DJ. The cyclic vomiting syndrome threshold: a framework for understanding pathogenesis and predicting successful treatments. Clin Transl Gastroenterol 2016;7(10):e198.

20. Gelfand AA, Gallagher RC. Cyclic vomiting syndrome versus inborn errors of metabolism: a review with clinical recommendations. Headache 2016;56(1):215–21.

21. Venkatesan T, Zadvornova Y, Raff H, et al. Endocannabinoid-related lipids are increased during an episode of cyclic vomiting syndrome. Neurogastroenterol Motil 2016;28(9):1409–18.
22. Venkatesan T, Levinthal DJ, Tarbell SE, et al. Guidelines on management of cyclic vomiting syndrome in adults by the American Neurogastroenterology and Motility Society and the Cyclic Vomiting Syndrome Association. Neurogastroenterol Motil 2019;31(Suppl 2):e13604.
23. Ruberto AJ, Sivilotti MLA, Forrester S, et al. Intravenous haloperidol versus on-dansetron for cannabis hyperemesis syndrome (HaVOC): a randomized, controlled trial. Ann Emerg Med 2020.
24. Lee C, Greene SL, Wong A. The utility of droperidol in the treatment of cannabi-noid hyperemesis syndrome. Clin Toxicol (Phila) 2019;57(9):773–7.
25. Mortimer MJ, Kay J, Jaron A. Clinical epidemiology of childhood abdominal migraine in an urban general practice. Dev Med Child Neurol 1993;35(3):243–8.
26. Abu-Arafeh I, Russell G. Prevalence and clinical features of abdominal migraine compared with those of migraine headache. Arch Dis Child 1995;72(5):413–7.
27. Karmali R, Hall-Wurst G. Fifty-eight-year-old female with abdominal migraine: a rare cause of episodic gastrointestinal disturbance in adults. Clin Case Rep 2020;8(8):1340–5.
28. Winner P. Abdominal migraine. Semin Pediatr Neurol 2016;23(1):11–3.
29. Rasquin A, Di Lorenzo C, Forbes D, et al. Childhood functional gastrointestinal disorders: child/adolescent. Gastroenterology 2006;130(5):1527–37.
30. Irwin S, Barmherzig R, Gelfand A. Recurrent gastrointestinal disturbance: abdominal migraine and cyclic vomiting syndrome. Curr Neurol Neurosci Rep 2017;17(3):21.
31. Mortimer MJ, Kay J, Jaron A, et al. Does a history of maternal migraine or depres-sion predispose children to headache and stomach-ache? Headache 1992; 32(7):353–5.
32. Mani J, Madani S. Pediatric abdominal migraine: current perspectives on a lesser known entity. Pediatr Health Med Ther 2018;9:47–58.
33. Napthali K, Koloski N, Talley NJ. Abdominal migraine. Cephalalgia 2016;36(10): 980–6.
34. Woodruff AE, Cieri NE, Abeles J, et al. Abdominal migraine in adults: a review of pharmacotherapeutic options. Ann Pharmacother 2013;47(6):e27.
35. Angus-Leppan H, Saatci D, Sutcliffe A, et al. Abdominal migraine. BMJ 2018;360: k179.
36. Hirsch W, Nee J, Ballou S, et al. Emergency department burden of gastroparesis in the United States, 2006-2013. J Clin Gastroenterol 2019;53(2):109–13.
37. Rey E, Choung RS, Schleck CD, et al. Prevalence of hidden gastroparesis in the community: the gastroparesis "iceberg". J Neurogastroenterol Motil 2012;18: 34–42.
38. Jung HK, Choung RS, Locke GR III, et al. The incidence, prevalence and survival of gastroparesis in Olmsted County, Minnesota 1996–2006. Gastroenterology 2008;134(Suppl 1):A534–5.
39. Parkman HP, Yates K, Hasler WL, et al. Similarities and differences between dia-betic and idiopathic gastroparesis. Clin Gastroenterol Hepatol 2011;9:1056–64.
40. Ye Y, Jiang B, Manne S, et al. Epidemiology and outcomes of gastroparesis, as documented in general practice records, in the United Kingdom. Gut 2020. gutjnl-2020-321277.
41. Grover M, Farrugia G, Stanghellini V. Gastroparesis: a turning point in under-standing and treatment. Gut 2019;68(12):2238–50.

42. Farrugia G. Histologic changes in diabetic gastroparesis. Gastroenterol Clin North Am 2015;44:31–8.
43. Camilleri M, Bharucha AE, Farrugia G. Epidemiology, mechanisms, and management of diabetic gastro- 6. paresis. Clin Gastroenterol Hepatol 2011;9(1):5–12.
44. Hasler WL, Wilson LA, Parkman HP, et al. Factors related to abdominal pain in gastroparesis: contrast to patients with predominant nausea and vomiting. Neurogastroenterol Motil 2013;25:427, e301.
45. Parkman HP, Yates K, Hasler WL, et al. National Institute of Diabetes and Digestive and Kidney Diseases Gastroparesis Clinical Research Consortium. Similarities and differences between diabetic and idiopathic gastroparesis. Clin Gastroenterol Hepatol 2011;9(12):1056–64.
46. Hasler WL. Gastroparesis. Curr Opin Gastroenterol 2012;28(6):621–8.
47. Parkman HP, Hasler WL, Fisher RS, et al. American gastroenterological association medical position statement: diagnosis and treatment of gastroparesis. Gastroenterology 2004;127:1589–91.
48. Metoclopramide. Lexidrugs. Hudson, OH: Lexicomp; 2021. Available at: http://online.lexi.com/. Accessed January 30, 2021.
49. Pittayanon R, Yuan Y, Bollegala NP, et al. Prokinetics for functional dyspepsia. Cochrane Database Syst Rev 2018;10(10):CD009431.
50. Roldan CJ, Chambers KA, Paniagua L, et al. Randomized controlled double-blind trial comparing haloperidol combined with conventional therapy to conventional therapy alone in patients with symptomatic gastroparesis. Acad Emerg Med 2017;24(11):1307–14.
51. Ramirez R, Stalcup P, Croft B, et al. Haloperidol undermining gastroparesis symptoms (HUGS) in the emergency department. Am J Emerg Med 2017; 35(8):1118–20.
52. van Nieuwenhoven MA, Vriens BE, Brummer RJ, et al. Effect of dehydration on gastrointestinal function at rest and during exercise in humans. Eur J Appl Physiol 2000;83(6):578–84.
53. Webster DR, Henrikson HW, Currie DJ. The effect of potassium deficiency on intestinal motility and gastric secretion. Ann Surg 1950;132(4):779–83.
54. Sperber AD, Bangdiwala SI, Drossman DA, et al. Worldwide prevalence and burden of functional gastrointestinal disorders, results of rome foundation global study. Gastroenterology 2021;160(1):99–114.e3.
55. Hungin AP, Chang L, Locke GR, et al. Irritable bowel syndrome in the United States: prevalence, symptom patterns and impact. Aliment Pharmacol Ther 2005;21(11):1365–75.
56. Ford AC, Talley NJ, Veldhuyzen van Zanten SJ, et al. Will the history and physical examination help establish that irritable bowel syndrome is causing this patient's lower gastrointestinal tract symptoms? [published correction appears in JAMA. 2009 Apr 15;301(15):1544]. JAMA 2008;300(15):1793–805.
57. Zhu Y, Zheng X, Cong Y, et al. Bloating and distention in irritable bowel syndrome: the role of gas production and visceral sensation after lactose ingestion in a population with lactase deficiency. Am J Gastroenterol 2013;108(9):1516–25.
58. American College of Gastroenterology Task Force on Irritable Bowel Syndrome, Brandt LJ, Chey WD, Foxx-Orenstein AE, et al. An evidence-based position statement on the management of irritable bowel syndrome. Am J Gastroenterol 2009; 104(Suppl 1):S1–35.
59. Hanevik K, Dizdar V, Langeland N, et al. Development of functional gastrointestinal disorders after Giardia lamblia infection. BMC Gastroenterol 2009;9:27.

60. Yang M, Zhang L, Hong G, et al. Duodenal and rectal mucosal microbiota related to small intestinal bacterial overgrowth in diarrhea-predominant irritable bowel syndrome. J Gastroenterol Hepatol 2020;35(5):795–805.
61. Kaptchuk TJ, Kelley JM, Conboy LA, et al. Components of placebo effect: randomised controlled trial in patients with irritable bowel syndrome. BMJ 2008; 336(7651):999–1003.
62. Sanders DS, Carter MJ, Hurlstone DP, et al. Association of adult coeliac disease with irritable bowel syndrome: a case-control study in patients fulfilling ROME II criteria referred to secondary care. Lancet 2001;358(9292):1504–8.
63. Plavšić I, Hauser G, Tkalčić M, et al. Diagnosis of irritable bowel syndrome: role of potential biomarkers. Gastroenterol Res Pract 2015;2015:490183.
64. Lu PL, Mousa HM. Constipation: beyond the old paradigms. Gastroenterol Clin North Am 2018;47(4):845–62.
65. Ford AC, Moayyedi P, Chey WD, et al. American College of Gastroenterology monograph on management of irritable bowel syndrome. Am J Gastroenterol 2018;113(Suppl 2):1–18.
66. Cotton PB, Elta GH, Carter CR, et al. Rome IV. Gallbladder and sphincter of oddi disorders. Gastroenterology 2016.
67. Behar J, Corazziari E, Guelrud M, et al. Functional gallbladder and sphincter of oddi disorders. Gastroenterology 2006;130(5):1498–509.
68. Richmond BK, DiBaise J, Ziessman H. Utilization of cholecystokinin cholescintigraphy in clinical practice. J Am Coll Surg 2013;217(2):317–23.
69. Bates JA, Dinnan K, Sharp V. Biliary hyperkinesia, a new diagnosis or misunderstood pathophysiology of dyskinesia: a case report. Int J Surg Case Rep 2019; 55:80–3.
70. Carr JA, Walls J, Bryan LJ, et al. The treatment of gallbladder dyskinesia based upon symptoms: results of a 2-year, prospective, nonrandomized, concurrent cohort study. Surg Laparosc Endosc Percutan Tech 2009;19(3):222–6.
71. Vegunta RK, Raso M, Pollock J, et al. Biliary dyskinesia: the most common indication for cholecystectomy in children. Surgery 2005;138(4):726–33.
72. Bielefeldt K. The rising tide of cholecystectomy for biliary dyskinesia. Aliment Pharmacol Ther 2013;37(1):98–106.
73. Whitehead WE, Palsson O, Jones KR. Systematic review of the comorbidity of irritable bowel syndrome with other disorders: what are the causes and implications? Gastroenterology 2002;122(4):1140–56.
74. Aggarwal N, Bielefeldt K. Diagnostic stringency and healthcare needs in patients with biliary dyskinesia. Dig Dis Sci 2013;58(10):2799–808.
75. Bielefeldt K. Gastroparesis: concepts, controversies, and challenges. Scientifica (Cairo) 2012;2012:424802.

UNITED STATES POSTAL SERVICE®
Statement of Ownership, Management, and Circulation
(All Periodicals Publications Except Requester Publications)

1. Publication Title	2. Publication Number	3. Filing Date
EMERGENCY MEDICINE CLINICS OF NORTH AMERICA	000 – 714	9/18/2021

4. Issue Frequency	5. Number of Issues Published Annually	6. Annual Subscription Price
FEB, MAY, AUG, NOV	4	$359.00

7. Complete Mailing Address of Known Office of Publication (Not printer) (Street, city, county, state, and ZIP+4®)

ELSEVIER INC.
230 Park Avenue, Suite 800
New York, NY 10169

Contact Person
Malathi Samayan

Telephone (Include area code)
91-44-4299-4507

8. Complete Mailing Address of Headquarters or General Business Office of Publisher (Not printer)

ELSEVIER INC.
230 Park Avenue, Suite 800
New York, NY 10169

9. Full Names and Complete Mailing Addresses of Publisher, Editor, and Managing Editor (Do not leave blank)

Publisher (Name and complete mailing address)

Dolores Meloni, ELSEVIER INC.
1600 JOHN F KENNEDY BLVD. SUITE 1800
PHILADELPHIA, PA 19103-2899

Editor (Name and complete mailing address)

JOANNA COLLETT, ELSEVIER INC.
1600 JOHN F KENNEDY BLVD. SUITE 1800
PHILADELPHIA, PA 19103-2899

Managing Editor (Name and complete mailing address)

PATRICK MANLEY, ELSEVIER INC.
1600 JOHN F KENNEDY BLVD. SUITE 1800
PHILADELPHIA, PA 19103-2899

10. Owner (Do not leave blank. If the publication is owned by a corporation, give the name and address of the corporation immediately followed by the names and addresses of all stockholders owning or holding 1 percent or more of the total amount of stock. If not owned by a corporation, give the names and addresses of the individual owners. If owned by a partnership or other unincorporated firm, give its name and address as well as those of each individual owner. If the publication is published by a nonprofit organization, give its name and address.)

Full Name	Complete Mailing Address
WHOLLY OWNED SUBSIDIARY OF REED/ELSEVIER, US HOLDINGS	1600 JOHN F KENNEDY BLVD. SUITE 1800 PHILADELPHIA, PA 19103-2899

11. Known Bondholders, Mortgagees, and Other Security Holders Owning or Holding 1 Percent or More of Total Amount of Bonds, Mortgages, or Other Securities. If none, check box ▶ ☐ None

Full Name	Complete Mailing Address
N/A	

12. Tax Status (For completion by nonprofit organizations authorized to mail at nonprofit rates) (Check one)
The purpose, function, and nonprofit status of this organization and the exempt status for federal income tax purposes:
☒ Has Not Changed During Preceding 12 Months
☐ Has Changed During Preceding 12 Months (Publisher must submit explanation of change with this statement)

PS Form **3526**, July 2014 (Page 1 of 4 (see instructions page 4)) PSN: 7530-01-000-9931 PRIVACY NOTICE: See our privacy policy on www.usps.com.

---

13. Publication Title	14. Issue Date for Circulation Data Below
EMERGENCY MEDICINE CLINICS OF NORTH AMERICA	MAY 2021

15. Extent and Nature of Circulation			Average No. Copies Each Issue During Preceding 12 Months	No. Copies of Single Issue Published Nearest to Filing Date
a. Total Number of Copies (Net press run)			250	219
b. Paid Circulation (By Mail and Outside the Mail)	(1)	Mailed Outside-County Paid Subscriptions Stated on PS Form 3541 (Include paid distribution above nominal rate, advertiser's proof copies, and exchange copies)	136	84
	(2)	Mailed In-County Paid Subscriptions Stated on PS Form 3541 (Include paid distribution above nominal rate, advertiser's proof copies, and exchange copies)	0	0
	(3)	Paid Distribution Outside the Mails Including Sales Through Dealers and Carriers, Street Vendors, Counter Sales, and Other Paid Distribution Outside USPS®	58	53
	(4)	Paid Distribution by Other Classes of Mail Through the USPS (e.g. First-Class Mail®)	0	0
c. Total Paid Distribution (Sum of 15b (1), (2), (3), and (4))		▶	194	137
d. Free or Nominal Rate Distribution (By Mail and Outside the Mail)	(1)	Free or Nominal Rate Outside-County Copies included on PS Form 3541	39	65
	(2)	Free or Nominal Rate In-County Copies Included on PS Form 3541	0	0
	(3)	Free or Nominal Rate Copies Mailed at Other Classes Through the USPS (e.g. First-Class Mail)	0	0
	(4)	Free or Nominal Rate Distribution Outside the Mail (Carriers or other means)	0	0
e. Total Free or Nominal Rate Distribution (Sum of 15d (1), (2), (3) and (4))		▶	39	65
f. Total Distribution (Sum of 15c and 15e)		▶	233	202
g. Copies not Distributed (See Instructions to Publishers #4 (page 3))		▶	17	17
h. Total (Sum of 15f and g)		▶	250	219
i. Percent Paid (15c divided by 15f times 100)			83.26%	67.82%

* If you are claiming electronic copies, go to line 16 on page 3. If you are not claiming electronic copies, skip to line 17 on page 3.

16. Electronic Copy Circulation		Average No. Copies Each Issue During Preceding 12 Months	No. Copies of Single Issue Published Nearest to Filing Date
a. Paid Electronic Copies	▶		
b. Total Paid Print Copies (Line 15c) + Paid Electronic Copies (Line 16a)	▶		
c. Total Print Distribution (Line 15f) + Paid Electronic Copies (Line 16a)	▶		
d. Percent Paid (Both Print & Electronic Copies) (16b divided by 16c × 100)	▶		

☒ I certify that 50% of all my distributed copies (electronic and print) are paid above a nominal price.

17. Publication of Statement of Ownership

☒ If the publication is a general publication, publication of this statement is required. Will be printed in the NOVEMBER 2021 issue of this publication. ☐ Publication not required.

18. Signature and Title of Editor, Publisher, Business Manager, or Owner

Malathi Samayan - Distribution Controller

Malathi Samayan

Date 9/18/2021

I certify that all information furnished on this form is true and complete. I understand that anyone who furnishes false or misleading information on this form or who omits material or information requested on the form may be subject to criminal sanctions (including fines and imprisonment) and/or civil sanctions (including civil penalties).

PS Form **3526**, July 2014 (Page 3 of 4) PRIVACY NOTICE: See our privacy policy on www.usps.com.

Printed and bound by CPI Group (UK) Ltd, Croydon, CR0 4YY

08/05/2025

01864704-0004